"If there is one thing I know having worked with hundreds of doctors every year for more than two decades, it's that most of them are all talk and no action. If you want someone who is the real deal to be your guide on your journey to the life you deserve through oral health, then look no further than Dr. Robert Herzog. A passionate, humorous, loving, family man and masterful clinician, the best part of Dr. Herzog is he loves what he does and follows all the advice he is dishing out here in this book. In fact, it is his own health journey that motivated him to do more to share, educate, and ultimately, help his patients throughout the country.

Having known Dr. Herzog personally for several years, there is no one who I would trust more and want to be the leader of my family's health more so than him. You'll get a lot out of this book—it will be enlightening, inspirational, and eye-opening. But if you want Dr. Herzog to deliver the goods on a better you, the best way is to convince him to become your doctor. That's when the real magic happens. And there's nothing better you could do to give yourself an advantage on your future than this. You are in the right place at the right time. Read this book now, just don't stop there. Take action. Because that is exactly what Dr. Herzog has done his whole life: continual learning, discovering, and passionate, committed action. Enjoy your journey to better health! You deserve it, just ask Dr. Herzog!"

Scott Manning, MBA

"As an integrative physician I am naturally drawn to biologic dentistry for my family's dental care. Both of these holistic approaches to healthcare share the basic tenets of patient-centered care that seeks to apply the best of conventional and complementary therapies for safe and effective results, nurture intrinsic healing, and honor the therapeutic relationship. Dr. Herzog's open-minded and expansive approach to his calling is evident in this book, and he gives testimony to the fact that biologic dentistry isn't a new specialty, rather, it is just good dentistry."

Ann Carey Tobin, MD, FAAFP

"Dr. Herzog has hit a home run with this text. He describes biologic dentistry in a commonsense way we can all understand. Dr. Herzog is a gifted clinician and educator, as he aptly describes biologic dentistry as truly a humanistic approach to overall health and wellness. This important text should be read by every physician and traditional dentist with an open mind. The result will be much improved outcomes for their patients."

Phil Mollica, MS, DMD, NMD, IBDM, MIAOMT, FAAOT

Doctor of Integrative Medicine
President, Professor
American College of Integrative Medicine and Dentistry
School of Integrative Biologic Dental Medicine
President, American Academy of Ozonetherapy

BIOLOGIC DENTISTRY

AND A BETTER YOU

BIOLOGIC DENTISTRY
AND A BETTER YOU

ORAL CARE'S CONNECTION TO OVERALL BODY HEALTH

ROBERT HERZOG, DDS, FAGD
WITH BUD RAMEY

Advantage | Books

Published by Advantage, Charleston, South Carolina.
Member of Advantage Media.

ADVANTAGE is a registered trademark, and the Advantage colophon is a trademark of Advantage Media Group, Inc.

Printed in the United States of America.

10 9 8 7 6 5 4 3 2 1

ISBN: 978-1-64225-709-0 (Paperback)
ISBN: 978-1-64225-708-3 (eBook)

LCCN: 2023906272

Cover design by Danna Steele.
Layout design by Wesley Strickland.

This publication is designed to provide accurate and authoritative information in regard to the subject matter covered. It is sold with the understanding that the publisher is not engaged in rendering legal, accounting, or other professional services. If legal advice or other expert assistance is required, the services of a competent professional person should be sought.

This book contains the opinions and ideas of the author(s). It is intended to provide informative material in a general nature on the subjects in the publication. As such it is not in any way a substitute for the advice of the readers own dentist, physician or other medical professional based on the reader's own individual conditions, symptoms, or concerns. If the reader needs personal medical, health, dietary, exercise, or other assistance or advice, the reader should consult a competent dentist, physician, and/or other qualified health care professional. The author(s) specifically disclaim all responsibility for injury, damage, loss or risk, personal or otherwise, which is incurred as a direct or indirect consequence of following any directions or suggestions or use and application of any of the contents of this book.

Advantage Media helps busy entrepreneurs, CEOs, and leaders write and publish a book to grow their business and become the authority in their field. Advantage authors comprise an exclusive community of industry professionals, idea-makers, and thought leaders. Do you have a book idea or manuscript for consideration? We would love to hear from you at **AdvantageMedia.com**.

This book is dedicated to fellow travelers
in search of health solutions.

Two roads diverged in a wood, and I—
I took the one less traveled by,
And that made all the difference.

—ROBERT FROST

ACKNOWLEDGMENTS

I want to thank all the people who helped transform me into the person I am today.

Mom and Dad—guiding lights and shapers of my potential, always believing in me. Thank you.

My family. Susan, Luke, Brian, and Eric—the core. We have braved through the challenges and celebrated the many successes. Through each of you I have grown to be a better person, husband, and father. Love you all.

Kathy—office confidant and right-hand colleague. My respect for your intuition and wisdom, which has helped guide my career from novice dentist to skilled practitioner, is beyond words. Your dedication has given life to our practice. Its success is heavily due to you. I will always be grateful.

Bud—my writing coach. What a fun adventure we had writing this book. A debt of gratitude for your help with the storytelling process. You are an all-star!

My family, friends, colleagues, staff, and supporters of my career decisions over the years. Each one of you provided guidance and encouragement along the many paths. Be well and stay well. Thank you.

Forbes Books, my publisher. Thank you for a great experience from beginning to end, as well as a national platform upon which to share my story.

ROBERT HERZOG DDS, FAGD

Dr. Robert Herzog's wife, Susan, best describes why he developed *Biologic Dentistry and a Better You.*

"Rob has spent years devoting every waking moment to practicing dentistry that is more holistic, safe, and friendly to the body," Susan noted.

As this book began to develop, she asked him, "Will you be writing your book for dentists, doctors, or patients?"

Dr. Herzog reflected, "It's for my patients … and anyone who wants a closer look at this new world of dentistry."

Dr. Herzog prepared this narrative for people who feel curious about the "coming of age" of such topics as holistic extractions, holistic root canals, dental meridians; the use of ozone, lasers, and 3D x-rays in dentistry; and lymphatic systems, sleep issues, and the potential toxic risks of fluoride, mercury, and amalgam. *Holistic dentistry* prevents and treats disease and helps maintain oral health using natural therapies, safely.

Robert Herzog, DDS, has practiced in Albany, New York, for over a quarter century, constantly advancing and curating the world's newest holistic and biologic dental practices. Deeply rooted in dental tradition, he began his career as an electrical engineer, a profession of problem solvers. When he instead decided to become a dentist, he deployed that talent to solving health problems for his patients, deploying carefully selected new ones and advanced practices of *biologic dentistry*.

A *biologic dentist* will assess the patient's entire state of physical and emotional health before deciding on treatments, is always ambitious about safety, and is often very open-minded.

"The body is an interconnected system. When something isn't right, it often shows up in the mouth," Dr. Herzog observes. "So, we can get to the root of systemic problems by starting with the mouth."

CONTENTS

PREFACE

This Book Will Spark Your Curiosity about the Mouth-Body Connection

Our culture has changed the way we communicate. The information resides at our fingertips, so much so that it has become difficult to sort out and find true evidence-based healthcare information. Most folks can acquire the research, but it often needs interpretation. Much of modern medicine has a repressed past, not to be reviewed or recalled. If we go there, we might bring back unwanted artifacts.

We know we can trust evidence-based medicine such as Class I, placebo-controlled, double-blind clinical trials. But new and exciting protocols and technologies emerge daily in medicine and dentistry. The media devotes more bandwidth to these topics than ever before. Many people now lend credence to ideas once considered fringe issues and theories. As this cultural reprocessing continues, twenty-first-century healthcare consumers have reached a tipping point regarding holistic medicine, a trend I applaud. It's clinical decision-making without background noise.

Biologic dentistry should not be viewed as a separate, recognized specialty of dentistry but as an open-minded, disciplined thought process that always seeks the safest, least toxic way to accomplish modern dentistry and contemporary healthcare goals. The tenets of biologic dentistry can inform and intersect with all topics of conversation in healthcare, as the mouth's well-being plays an integral role in the health of the whole person.

Many sick and frustrated patients come into my office for their initial visit, looking for answers. Some have tried several healthcare professionals but still don't have the answers they need to feel better and function as healthy people. And often, they do not know what questions to ask.

Decades back, when the only restorative materials were amalgam or gold, and the only aesthetic material was denture teeth, our profession had limited options to fulfill its mission and be biologically discriminating simultaneously. Today, we can do better—less toxic, more individualized, and more environmentally friendly than ever. Not only do we realize that physical conditions like poor nutrition and smoking have a tangible impact on oral health, but we have also concluded that poor oral health has been linked to conditions such as heart disease, diabetes, Alzheimer's, and complications during pregnancy.

AS A TRADITIONAL, HOLISTIC/BIOLOGIC, AND WELLNESS OFFICE, WE PROVIDE PATIENTS WITH THE INFORMATION THEY NEED TO MAKE THE BEST AND MOST INFORMED CHOICES ABOUT ORAL HEALTHCARE.

As a traditional, holistic/biologic, and wellness office, we provide patients with the information they need to make the best and most informed choices about oral healthcare. This includes both conventional and biological options. We customize our treatments by combining the best of modern dentistry and complementary therapies. This approach works well for all our patients and is particularly helpful for people with complex dental problems, chronic health issues, or a combination of both.

As it always has been, a long-term relationship with every patient forms the basis for success. The more we learn about the body, the more remarkably intertwined it becomes.

In your community, you may encounter dental practitioners who use the phrase *holistic dentistry* or *biologic dentistry*. *Holistic dentistry* describes the practice of diagnosing, preventing, treating, and maintaining oral health using natural therapies. *Biologic dentistry* assesses a patient's entire state of physical and emotional health before deciding on treatments. It fascinates me that after using these safer, more holistic practices for years, I can spend just a few minutes with a new patient and almost immediately begin to see a connection. The lights go on when you view the entire body as a singular unit, not just the mouth. Some of it may be intuition, but I doubt it. I am a pragmatic engineer. I solve problems. I go about it in a wider lane than most general dentists.

I would never try to be a medical doctor. But I find that being a member of the patient's team and collaborating with the patient's MD and other providers makes the sum more significant than all the parts.

In *Biologic Dentistry and a Better You*, I will explain the complex science behind issues in the mouth and how they affect the whole body—and vice versa. Through stories and case studies, you will learn more about the mouth-body connection, dental meridians, different metals, safe extractions, TMJ (clenching) and sleep, detoxifying the brain, and inflammation and gut health. We will review treatments (only those in which I have developed great confidence) that combine Eastern and Western medicine to make patients smile and their whole body healthier and happier.

Biologic dentistry also carefully considers the whole-body effects of all dental materials, techniques, and procedures, new and old. Most practices create a fluoride-free, mercury-free, and mercury-safe environment. Individualized testing for the biocompatibility of dental materials employs another close look at safety. Biologic dentists insist that all clinical practices use components that sustain life or improve the patient's quality of life.

The word "biologic" refers to life. In some ways, biologic dentistry could be considered conservative in that we typically guide our work to be minimally invasive yet appropriately proactive. When you speak with a biologic dentist, you will instantly see what we understand with absolute certainty: that the complex, dynamic relationships of oral and systemic health within the context of the whole person are inseparable.

In using the term *biologic*, we do not attempt to stake out a new specialty for dentistry but rather to describe a philosophy that can apply to all facets of dental practice and healthcare in general: always seek the safest, least toxic way to accomplish the mission of treatment, all the goals of modern dentistry, and do it while treading as lightly as possible on the patient's biological terrain—a more biocompatible approach to oral health.

I offer you this view of the emerging field of *holistic* and biologic dentistry through my experiences and problem-solving findings. I have rigorously curated the best for you under the bright light of this stubborn, pragmatic engineer/dentist who believes deeply that the mouth is a window to whole body health. There is an earthy authenticity to it all. Today, we both have front-row seats.

PROLOGUE

The Pace of Innovation

There are reasons biologic dentistry grows in popularity. We reside in a population of people making new discoveries about health and prevention every day.

And general dentistry as a whole has made great strides in these last two decades, advancements that have benefited everyone in the nation.

In late 2021, a long-awaited report was issued offering a comprehensive summary of those advances. The National Institute of Dental and Craniofacial Research (NIDCR) published the first such report in more than twenty years titled *Oral Health in America: Advances and Challenges.*

This lengthy study resulted from two years of research and writing by over four hundred contributors. As a follow-up to the *Surgeon General's Report on Oral Health in America,* this body of work explores the nation's oral health over the last twenty years.[1]

---

1   "Oral Health in America," https://www.nidcr.nih.gov/ (National Institute of Dental and Craniofacial Research, 2021).

A well-written stroll down memory lane, this report enlightens both for what the authors mention and what they do not mention. Dentistry races through time with continual advancements in every aspect of practice, with notable advances affecting oral health in America since 2000.

Since the Year 2000

IMPACT OF SEALANTS

The expanded use of dental sealants, an important cavity prevention service, has led to meaningful reductions of some oral health disparities by race/ethnicity and income for many children.

TOOTH LOSS IMPROVING

Tooth loss continues to decline across all subgroups of adults. Among adults aged sixty-five to seventy-four years, only 13 percent are edentulous (lacking teeth), compared with 50 percent in the 1960s.

ADVANCED DENTAL MATERIALS

Impressive progress has been made in how we provide care—from the use of advanced dental materials to restoring the form and function of the teeth (dentition) when filling a cavity, making crowns, and replacing missing teeth—to diagnosing, treatment planning, and managing oral pain.

IMPLANTS

There has been a fourfold increase in the percentage of older adults receiving dental implants during the last twenty years. Major advances in implant technology and practice have made placing implants faster and more successful than ever before, improving the quality of life for many. Unfortunately, implant procedures remain costly and, therefore, out of reach for most adults.

A Better Understanding of Our Microbiome

We now have a better understanding of the microbiome. (The bacteria, fungi, and viruses that live in our mouths make up the oral microbiome.) This term describes the community of microbes—both beneficial and harmful—that inhabit our bodies. In-depth knowledge of the oral microbiome moves us closer to the promise of personalized oral healthcare, in which specific microbial therapies can be individually developed to prevent, manage, and treat oral diseases.[2]

---

2   Ibid.

PROPELLED BY DESPERATION INTO BIOLOGIC DENTISTRY

The Mouth-Body Connection

I have always enjoyed learning about the new holistic alternatives in medicine and dentistry. But that interest became a calling. My personal choice to study and later become an expert in biologic dental medicine was propelled by agitation, worry, and, finally, desperation.

The year was 2009. Something went terribly wrong with my eleven-year-old son, and we could not figure it out. One day, Brian came down with this mysterious headache, and it was excruciating. We first went to his pediatrician and, later, to a pediatric neurologist.

They were all saying, *Oh, I'm not sure what it is. Maybe he's clenching and maybe grinding.* Frustrated by that, my reaction was *Dude, I'm the dentist. I would know that.*

Maybe he has this or that. It kept going on and on and on. We wound up going to the Boston Children's Hospital, a magnet for excellence and among the most advanced pediatric hospitals in the nation. The baffling question: *Why did he have a persistent headache?* His pain continued. I tried to figure this out with the pediatricians, but nobody offered us answers. Brian had normal MRIs; the doctors were puzzled. They said he would *have to live with it.* No theories emerged. The diagnostic team put him on anti-seizure medicine, which ended up being very unpleasant and started to alter his personality. (We chose homeschooling for his seventh grade because he could not function in the school setting. He had to be tutored at home.)

A headache? A headache that never goes away, and then potentially, he will have to live with it. And I will tell you what: my frustration level climbed pretty high at that point. I thought, *Now we give up?* No. Solutions exist for these things. There may exist solutions other than the standard protocols. Whatever your training, if you get stumped, maybe somebody else can suggest a solution. I will never cede the field and walk off to the showers in the middle of a game. I will grapple with the problem and be a part of finding the solution. Yet I know we need to grade ourselves on a forgiving curve. No medical generation in history has traveled this far.

And if it is your kid, you will go anywhere to find an answer. Here is a boy who has been told to live with a terrible, intractable headache every day of his life until it "goes away." You can hope, but you still have a headache. You are undiagnosed, and your symptoms are subclinical. Well, what could that be? *You're a teenage boy … too much candy?*

Come on, docs, I live in the same household. I know what he's doing or not doing.

More and more imaging. More and more doctors. No answers.

So with Brian's condition, my open mind kicked into full gear. *There's something wrong here. Unshakable intuition. Informed intuition.*

I solve problems. Something seems amiss, elusive, cloaked. The secret code has not yet been cracked.

"*Grapple with the question.*"

Brian's symptoms got worse, and a new kind of dread set in. Then, just as our frustration level reached warp speed, Jennifer Goldstock, NP, a nurse practitioner caring for my son, weighed in. Lyme disease had just started peeking out from obscurity on the east coast. She suggested that she knew patients with an issue with Lyme disease, as she was also working with a Lyme doctor, Dr. Ronald Stram.

One of the nation's most prominent specialists in Lyme disease had an office in my hometown. We must be living right. Maybe that's it. Lyme disease, at that time, did not blink or beep on the radar screen of most physicians and triage in most emergency and urgent care settings. The symptoms were elusive and variable, and diagnosticians rarely rang the Lyme disease bell. Testing for the disease was just plain incomplete (and still needs work). Doctors debated how to treat the condition. (Even today, estimates reveal that 60 percent of people living with Lyme disease go undiagnosed in America.[3])

Dr. Ronald Stram and Jennifer Goldstock, NP, rang the bell.

"*Integrative medicine honors the physician-patient relationship, nurtures this partnership, and empowers the healer within.*"

—RONALD STRAM, MD, FACEP

---

3   Lisa A. Waddell et al., "The Accuracy of Diagnostic Tests for Lyme Disease in Humans, a Systematic Review and Meta-Analysis of North American Research," https://www.ncbi.nlm.nih.gov/ (U.S. National Library of Medicine, December 21, 2016), https://www.ncbi.nlm.nih.gov/pmc/articles/PMC5176185/.

Ronald Stram, MD, FACEP

Dr. Stram had become an evangelist about Lyme and its associated diseases among an inattentive medical community.

"Lyme disease needs to be a part of every physician's differential diagnosis," Dr. Stram preached around the country at national Lyme disease events. He hit the nail on the head in a vital address:

"Without considering Lyme disease as the cause of the affliction, we send patients down a spiral path of unnecessary and potentially harmful treatments. The increasing trend of the Lyme disease epidemic has been ascribed to ineffective preventive measures and outdated and unreliable testing, which the providers are relying on for diagnosis."[4]

He dove into an oppositional current. He gave clinicians a fresh understanding of this terrible disease. Dr. Ronald Stram, a lone figure of confidence and hope, eloquently proclaimed it a public health crisis.

Dr. Stram's twenty-five years as an emergency medicine physician had prompted him to recognize the need for holistic and preventative care to reduce the debilitation associated with chronic disease often seen too late in the emergency setting.

He completed an Integrative Medicine fellowship program at the University of Arizona with Dr. Andrew Weil in 2001. After his two-year fellowship training, he established the Stram Center for Integrative Medicine in 2003.

"More minds working as a team … has proved to be more effective in addressing the needs of patients."[5]

—DR. RONALD STRAM

---

4   Ibid.

5   Stram Center for Integrative Medicine, "Lyme Disease Education Forum," Stramcenter.com/services/lyme-disease/, accessed August 7, 2022.

The Stram Center's collaboration between conventionally trained medical doctors with complementary providers shows respect for wisdom and science across shared disciplines. More minds working as a team have proved to be more effective in addressing the needs of patients. His integrative approach reinforces my belief that healing can occur when a medical environment focuses on the social, emotional, physical, and spiritual needs of individuals with chronic health conditions and their support network.

Bittersweet Resolution

And that's when we began the road to recovery. It took an integrative medicine-trained physician to figure out a bittersweet resolution. Too much time had passed in clinical hibernation. Too much time had passed for patients looking for a diagnosis. Too much time passed for patients and parents being deflected from doctor to doctor, and my son, like so many others, walked around with these deadly bacteria slowly eroding his health.

Dr. Stram figured out that Brian had undiagnosed Lyme disease; it also may not have been a coincidence that at about the same time, he had the flu vaccine and the H1N1 vaccine. Those three things, at the same time, put his body into stress mode, into an inflammatory response.

The Stram Center started his recovery plan, and nutrition played a big part in it. Antibiotics in 2010 were also a big part of it. Doctors inserted a PICC line. (Mayo Clinic defines a PICC line as follows: "a peripherally inserted central catheter is a long, thin tube that's inserted through a vein in your arm and passed through to the larger veins near your heart."[6])

Now I am a believer. Over the years, we would again visit Dr. Stram (and his team) not only for Brian, but for my sons Eric and Luke, and myself. He has cared for all of us with various health issues over the years. My family had the unfortunate genetics of poor detoxification pathways. Correcting this has worked wonders for all of us.

After years of integrating biologic protocols into my practice, I have noted that people come to my biologic dentistry practice for one of several reasons:

- Very health-conscious folks who wish to take advantage of the least toxic, safest care available. They want to get well and stay well. They like the idea of whole-body dentistry as complementary to maintaining health and youthfulness.

- Young adults who want to correct some dentistry placed in their youth. They have a holistic lifestyle, and they want to fix that problem.

- People who do not feel in top health and have become frustrated with not getting answers from traditional medicine.

- Sick people—who are sick of looking for answers. They have tried numerous healthcare professionals but still don't have the necessary solutions to feel better and function well. They may have heard about biologic dentistry, but they don't know what it is and want to know more. They have a systemic problem that has yet to be solved.

---

6   "Peripherally Inserted Central Catheter (PICC) Line," mayoclinic.org (Mayo Foundation for Medical Education and Research, July 22, 2021), https://www.mayoclinic.org/tests-procedures/picc-line/about/pac-20468748#:~:text=A%20PICC%20line%20gives%20your,smaller%20veins%20in%20your%20arms.

- Regular dentistry patients who read my reviews and they want to see me because they think I am a good dentist. I often discover some potential issues they did not know about.

I have always enjoyed learning about the new holistic alternatives in medicine and dentistry. But that interest became a calling. My personal choice to study, and later become an expert in biologic dental medicine, was propelled by agitation, worry, and finally, desperation.

THE POWER OF BIOLOGIC DENTISTRY

Very recently, my patient Wesley came in struggling with a long-standing, very uncomfortable nodule in his neck. His physicians did not share his concern about it.

It wasn't cancerous, but he knew that this problem had a potential connection to a root canal tooth on the lower side, and he came in because nobody would believe him. And he had emotional issues over this. The word *desperation* comes to mind.

He urged me to provide the cone beam CT scan or 3D scan.

Immediately, we found the periapical pathology at the root tip, and I discovered this with him, because I like to read my initial x-rays, my initial findings, with our patients. If there's a revelation, they see it for themselves.

We wound up extracting it, and immediately, while still in the chair, his neck issue resolved right then and there. I allowed myself a smile, but during the procedure, as I finished the cleaning of the extraction site, his tears of emotional release flowed. We lived a decisive moment together. It's why I practice whole-body dentistry.

An Open Mind

A couple of decades ago, from a conservative practitioner's point of view, *holistic* seemed like a foreign language. Doctors and dentists felt reluctant to be associated with being *holistic* because their thought process was, *I'm a traditionally based dentist; I'm based and rooted in science—no quackery for me.*

Everyone has a different health path for their issues. And I'm just one of those tools that can help people potentially find an answer that they're probably not getting anywhere else. People go down the pathways of traditional medicine and can't find somebody who has a different opinion or wants to step outside the guardrails. It's okay to step out. You have to think for yourself.

I have a nephew in medical school right now, and we are so proud of him. We had a discussion recently, and I offered him a straightforward piece of advice. I said, "Christopher, you have to learn what they teach you in school, but you need an open mind if you want to help your patients."

The Stram team sought a dentist who understood this Lyme piece and how the mouth relates to the body. So, I got hooked. We were all learning about this Lyme puzzle and how to help a patient overcome their Lyme issues concurrently. It always seemed like I followed two steps behind the physicians in my research, but I couldn't treat my son Brian medically, right? I used their information and resources and started thinking about the dental piece and how it could help.

During that time, I studied more about the dental implications of systemic issues and began to become a contributor to the growing community of Lyme researchers. Why do patients clench? Why do they have brain fog? Why are they grinding their teeth (called bruxing)? They may have detoxification pathway issues, and their brain does not clear. The glial system, something researchers have found in the last five years, enables our brain to clear itself nightly if we get good sleep. We did not even know we had this system.

The clinical journal *Neurochemical Research* describes the glymphatic system as a "recently discovered macroscopic waste clearance system to promote efficient elimination of soluble proteins and metabolites from the central nervous system."[7]

Intriguingly, the glymphatic system functions mainly during sleep and becomes largely disengaged during wakefulness. The physical need for sleep across all species may therefore reflect that the brain must enter a state of activity that enables the elimination of potentially neurotoxic waste products.

Recent studies also indicate a close relationship and significant pathology in neurodegenerative disorders, traumatic brain injury, and stroke.

THE POWER OF BIOLOGIC DENTISTRY

A gentleman came in. I had not seen Jim for years. When we did his history and physical, it turned out that he had other health issues. He experienced severe foot issues resulting in multiple gangrenous tissue removals from his feet and toes.

In the absence of systemic disease like diabetes, I looked at him and said, *Your oral condition is not conducive to healing.*

I convinced him to permit me to extract several unrestorable and abscessed teeth, and by doing so, the desired result took place. By removing the oral infections, his body had an easier time healing his foot infection, and he quickly healed up. And, of course, Jim came back a few months later to tell me this great news, and to have his dental checkup. We chuckled at the fact that his doctors were doing a victory lap. He knew that if we had not cleared up his mouth, this might never have happened.

---

7   Nadia Aalling Jessen et al., "The Glymphatic System: A Beginner's Guide," https://www.ncbi.nlm.nih.gov/ (U.S. National Library of Medicine, May 7, 2015), https://www.ncbi.nlm.nih.gov/pmc/articles/PMC4636982/.

So, sleep becomes a new player in this whole experience.

If people clench and gnash their teeth and they have a sleep apnea issue undiagnosed, dentistry can come together with general medicine.

Like all anguished parents who struggle with their child's mystery illness, I became so focused on my kids that I failed to notice my symptoms. I, too, had Lyme disease at the same time. I suspected I had it for years, but the tests did not show positive until my general practitioner spotted it a couple of years later. I went every year for my annual physical; my general practitioner called me one day and said, *You know, all those symptoms have finally showed Lyme positive.* The Stram Center had been caring for me as well. I wondered. *Well, did the tests themselves get better? Were they more sensitive to this?*

Some physicians figure two pills of doxycycline and you're cured because it's a bacterial infection, but Lyme disease manifests in much more insidious ways, not just as a bacterial infection. There are a lot of nasty co-infections that go with it, such as (the most common tick-borne diseases in the United States) babesiosis, anaplasmosis, ehrlichiosis, relapsing fever, tularemia, and Rocky Mountain spotted fever (RMSF). Diseases acquired together like this are called co-infections, and clinical charts show eighteen different diseases.[8]

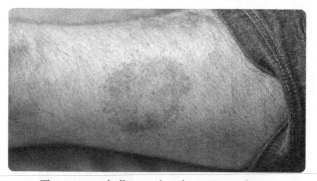

The signature bullseye rash indicates Lyme disease, but it does not always appear.

---

8   Lymedisease.org, "Other Lyme Disease Co-Infections," accessed August 27, 2022, https://www.lymedisease.org/lyme-basics/co-infections/other-co-infections/.

Of course, Brian didn't have the signature Lyme disease bullseye rash. Neither did I. But we have always enjoyed being a big scouting family. I took my boys on campouts every month. Could we have encountered Lyme disease-transmitting ticks there? I have no idea. Some of these ticks play a good game of hide-and-seek, so tiny that people get infected and never recall being bitten.

As stated previously, we eventually came to realize that Brian's body does not clear out toxins efficiently, an issue which was not understood then as well as it is today. All of these things, collectively, caused a bigger problem.

As part of my quest for deeper understanding, I joined the International Academy of Oral Medicine and Toxicology (IAOMT), a global network of dentists, health professionals, and scientists who research the biocompatibility of dental products, including the risks of mercury fillings, fluoride, root canals, and jawbone osteonecrosis. This group stays conservative enough for me, yet they take a lead in some of the most compelling topics in biologic dentistry. I can stand on their research and not be too far to the left or the right of mainstream dentistry. And then from there, their semiannual meetings opened my eyes because the participants talked about things that you don't see at a normal dental convention.

I learned about ozone dentistry, and I started incorporating that into my practice because it significantly reduces bacteria; it is a minimally invasive alternative that has the potential to ward off the advance of developing tooth decay, combined with other therapies.

And then I started thinking, from my past engineering work and what we learned a little bit about in dentistry, about how dissimilar metals cause issues in the mouth. It could be a problem if you have stainless steel crowns next to gold crowns, next to porcelain-fused-to-metal crowns, next to silver fillings (composed of half mercury, by the way), and next to titanium implants. Those all can cause a problem of dissimilar metals called *galvanism*.

And they're just like biting on a piece of tinfoil. When you were little, you may recall, if you had fillings in your mouth, biting on tin foil playfully might create these little microshocks. But today we understand that microshocks in an adult mouth do cause such an electrical disturbance field, and the disturbance field could be contributory to some issues. The brain resides inches away.

Next, improvements in dental imaging opened another door. I realized I had to get a 3D x-ray, a cone beam CAT scan x-ray, to look at infections because you cannot understand root canals and the hazards unless you can look at them with the 3D x-ray. The new 3D computed tomography (CT) is a scanning technology that allows us to view and inspect the external and internal structures of an object in 3D space. Computed tomography works by taking hundreds or thousands of 2D digital radiography projections around a 360-degree rotation of an object.

When I invested in that, I started finding undiagnosed infections in my patients, hiding under the tooth socket, invisible to standard dental x-rays.

And those infections potentially lay on a meridian, driving me to advance my understanding of that and study how that could contribute to their systemic nonwellness. It became a real adventure, like the feeling of hiking and exploring the wilderness. The energy meridians were first mapped and devised by Chinese medicine scholars over five thousand years ago. They are now commonly known as acupuncture meridians and acupressure points. Naturopathic medical schools and some conventional medical schools teach them. Tooth meridian charts are used by other medical specialists beyond holistic dentists, such as acupuncturists, naturopaths, functional doctors, and energy medicine practitioners.

THE POWER OF BIOLOGIC DENTISTRY

Early in my dental career, Mike came in with the whole right side of his face numb; the entire right side of his skin was numb from the top of his scalp down the back of his head.

I suspected a tooth and injected it with local anesthesia, a way I used to determine if it was a tooth problem or something else. I numbed an area I thought problematic—this was way before cone beam CT scans—and his pain disappeared.

His whole face resolved through that particular tooth that I knew was dead and needed a root canal, and within hours, his face resolved, the numbness completely gone.

After dental school, I furthered my education. I took advantage of an opportunity to study naturopathic medicine. Naturopathic medicine uses natural remedies to help the body heal itself. It embraces various therapies, including herbs, massage, acupuncture, exercise, and nutritional counseling. I have become board certified as a naturopathic physician and integrative biologic dental medicine.

That became a revelation. I did my research project on the effects of electromagnetic fields and the potential for harm to the human body, primarily because of my background as an electrical engineer. For me, everything relates to my engineering skills. Everything.

"A dentist is not the physician."

But I'm still a traditional dentist, and you have to understand that I work every day as a traditional dentist. I do standards of care as a traditional dentist, but I do more. I'm good at problem-solving and working with the patient and their team in helping to find answers to their illnesses, especially from my dental point of view. As an engineer, we're trained in problem-solving; we're trained in finding solutions. But a dentist is not a physician, so more and more, I began to collaborate with my patients' physicians. I knew that I needed a team, as a dentist probably will not be equipped to solve systemic problems alone.

I'm not a licensed naturopath in the state of New York because it's not recognized, but I deploy my education and work well with the patient's team. For an individual patient, this team might include a chiropractor, naturopath, nutritionist, and/or an acupuncturist. They'll also have their physician. We work collectively, and I provide dental information.

Do they have infections in their mouth? Did they have dissimilar metals? Could there exist a potential problem on a meridian that affects an organ? Do they have sleep issues? Are they tongue-tied, or is their palate too narrow for their tongue, and they clench at night? Do they breathe well? Dentists don't diagnose sleep apnea, by the way, but we make referrals for such disorders.

Another "Difficult Diagnostic Dilemma"[9]

DR. PAUL GRUNDY, THE GODFATHER OF THE PATIENT-CENTERED MEDICAL HOME

Dr. Paul Grundy, the international champion of primary care, describes a *trusted healer's* top responsibilities as solving "difficult diagnostic dilemmas" and cultivating personal relationships with patients. Dr. Grundy has traveled the world for IBM and now Innovaccer, urging primary care doctors to focus on diagnostics and patient relationships,

---

9   "Paul Grundy, MD, MPH, FACOEM, FACPM (Primary Care)," https://gtmr.org/ (Get the Medications Right, July 6, 2020), https://gtmr.org/team/paul-grundy-md-mph-facoem-facpm-primary-care/.

become *trusted healers,* and let the office team handle all the medical record entries, red tape, and paperwork.

My integrative medicine credentials have matured quite a bit since we first faced the crisis with Brian. That experience raised my radar, and I became much more open-minded to different modalities in order to come to a resolution. For my patients, and later with my family, I had a wider lane to maneuver.

And the next family crisis happened to my youngest son Eric after he had a vaccine injection booster to enter middle school. His hands went into contracture, and his elbows would not straighten out. The physicians wanted to start him on a lifetime biologic medicine (some of those things you read or hear about on TV) for juvenile rheumatoid arthritis.

This time, I no longer struggled like the rest of my fellow mystery-illness parents, without any complementary medicine options and alternatives. I approached Eric's condition with an open-minded view and a much bigger playing field. I woke up in the morning wanting to solve this active mystery.

What caused my son Eric to have this crisis? We quickly ruled out Lyme disease. I have a network of global alternative medicine colleagues, an intellectual brain trust in which we share expertise and advice. We had active discussions for weeks.

Doctors diagnosed him with juvenile rheumatoid arthritis. And again, you can be given a label like that, or like fibromyalgia, *but Doc, what do you do for that?*

And if you start on that medicine, you are probably on it for life. Did I want to put my eleven-year-old on that medicine? *No.* I decided to do it a different way, and he's remarkably better. Does he have flare-ups? He has flare-ups based on a sixteen-year-old kid having a diet binge, you know?

The important thing is that we did not want to live with this, and so we became an advocate for ourselves and our child, and we tried to find an alternative. I would say to parents that if you have a "difficult diagnostic dilemma," it's okay to be aggressive. Always be respectful, but pursue seeing other doctors. Passive acceptance will take you to a universe where problems fester.

My wife Susan kept an open mind for the treatments. (I think you would have to because we didn't go strictly down Main Street, so to speak.) But you must understand, after you've been married for all these years, when one spouse has strength, the other spouse honors that, and you run with it. Susan does not have the advanced medical connection or decades of continuous medical and engineering study. Still, she kept believing, knowing we have the best interest of our children in mind.

We avoided doing things that would be considered too extreme, and we always questioned our actions along the way, weighing our decision-making for treatment options. Do we go back to mainstream medicine? Does he need that 100 percent, or can we continue down an alternative path? And it took a little faith to go down the lesser-known journey of nontraditional medicine.

Susan feels my passion for holistic care, and she respects that I've spent all these years problem-solving, studying, reading, keeping an open mind, and not veering off too far left or right. But having that open-mindedness and then coming to some conclusion, a decision, and acting on it using a different tool—she respects that, too.

Almost at once, we observed more systemic reactions in Eric's condition as more and more symptoms arose. I concluded that his detoxification pathway was not proper. This became a difficult diagnostic dilemma, and our strategy was to deploy alternative therapies for Eric. We packed up and went to consult Jerry Tennant, MD,

MD(H), in Irving, Texas, who had become an international authority on healing through "energy medicine." Dr. Tennant and I had met at a national conference. Now we became patients of the Tennant Institute.

His "energy medicine" team has blended deep knowledge of Eastern and Western medicine and has developed special FDA-accepted tools. Dr. Tennant designed his BioModulator and Tennant BioTransducer with an eye on restoring and maintaining health. While twenty years ago I might have shaken off that idea, between my electrical engineering background and my growing understanding of the body's meridians and energy fields, we willingly adopted the advanced Tennant protocols with energy modalities. We tried pulse electromagnetic field therapies (PEMF) and light therapy (photo biomodulation), and we brought these into our home. Not surprisingly, these therapies work because they trigger specific repair activities within the body. The currents induced in tissues by PEMF mimic the natural electrical activities created within bones during movements.

Along with better nutrition, Eric made tremendous strides. Today, he functions just fine. His fingers are not in contractures anymore. I would say he continues to improve and now enjoys better than 90 percent of full recovery.

THE POWER OF BIOLOGIC DENTISTRY

Carl presented with transient brain cloud, difficulty concentrating, and on his right side, a dull pain.

He had very old fillings. Carl agreed to complete amalgam removal. Those teeth had fillings in them for thirty years or more, which means after that time frame, they do fail, break down, or develop fractures. It was a wise decision to do this. And after we finished, within hours, he experienced a relief he had not felt in years.

Many patients, after I extracted undiagnosed tooth pathology or infection by using the 3D x-ray, reported more energy, their gut got better, and their stomach issues became more manageable because infected teeth had been leaking toxins into the bloodstream.

Another patient suffered from facial pain and was diagnosed and put on medicine for neuropathy. It turned out to be a tooth issue. We find this stuff all the time.

Years after our Lyme disease nightmares, I still have residual symptoms from my Lyme disease. Because my Lyme testing took years to show positive, I now have lingering "long Lyme." When our medical system fails to diagnose and treat Lyme disease early, the spirochetes can spread and may go into hiding in different parts of the body. Weeks, months, or even years later, patients may develop problems with the brain and nervous system, muscles and joints, heart and circulation, digestion, reproductive system, and skin. Symptoms may disappear even without treatment, and different symptoms may appear at different times.[10]

I now know that if I have good body detoxification and elimination pathways, a good diet, stay healthy, and maintain a good exercise regimen, then my body can adapt to it. But I know when Lyme acts up in my body. When I have a challenge, I feel it from my waist down to my legs. I know. I waited too long to get care.

And in my experience, people can have cognitive function issues because of Lyme disease, such as brain fog or lingering malaise, and they just cannot figure things out. They can't concentrate. They can't read. They've had it for a long time. And it's very difficult to cross through the blood-brain barrier to help eradicate the problem.

---

10   Lymedisease.org, "Chronic Lyme Disease," Lymedisease.org, accessed August 14, 2022, https://www.lymedisease.org/lyme-basics/lyme-disease/chronic-lyme-disease/.

And that's where somebody like me can help, potentially, because people clench when they have those issues. And I have alternative treatment modalities.

Their body tries to eliminate it, but then they clench so much that they block the natural pathways of the glial system. It's helpful to have a doctor that has had that exposure to Lyme disease and won't just dismiss a patient's concerns. Unfortunately, a lot of Lyme patients have been told by their doctors that there is no such thing as *chronic Lyme.* However, it's becoming documented now in diagnostic codes for physicians, and ideally, that will help identify Lyme before it gets really bad.

We do not know exactly what percentage of diagnosed and treated people remain ill, but the CDC estimates up to 20 percent. A recent study of early Lyme disease reported that up to 36 percent remain ill.[11]

The reluctance of the diagnostic community to recognize *persistent Lyme* (or *chronic Lyme,* or *long Lyme)* has been mitigated by the recent open acceptance of *long Covid* disease. While one is a virus (COVID-19), and one (Lyme) is caused by a bacterium, the Borrelia bacteria is no less insidious than a virus, as it involves not just Lyme disease: it brings along baggage in the form of a host of co-infections.

As a patient, you must find out all you can about where you reside on the Lyme disease spectrum. You can have it, it can linger, and it can come back later for another, perhaps more life-threatening medical crisis.

"I question traditional everything."

There is a school of thought now among biologic dentists that we cannot rule out the possibility that Lyme lingers in areas of your

11   Ibid.

mouth not being reached by blood flow. Those would include areas of root canals and potential osteonecrosis lesions. I'm not sure if Lyme disease can live in those anaerobic spaces of the jaw. But I am also not sure it cannot. We await data, evidence, and experience. But that neural Lyme, when it begins to affect the behavior and the brain, that's devastating, because people can become nonfunctional.

Even today, at the point of care (either primary care, urgent care, or emergency care), we are still missing up to 60 percent of acute cases of Lyme disease. Though we're talking with our elected representatives at every opportunity, there's still not enough noise being made.

"The current 'gold standard' diagnostic for Lyme disease is a two-tiered ELISA/Western Blot blood test measuring human antibodies against *Borrelia burgdorferi*. This diagnostic is an indirect measure of infection, detecting the body's immunologic response to infection rather than detecting the Lyme bacteria itself. It misses up to 60 percent of cases of early-stage Lyme disease, as it can take weeks for the body to develop measurable antibodies against the infection."[12]

A team at Tufts University School of Medicine thinks they may have a novel approach to filling the gaps in existing testing technologies. While current testing makes it difficult to diagnose reinfection or successful treatment, "the anti-phospholipid autoantibodies—because of their quick increase and quick resolution with treatment—can fill these gaps as a novel additional test.

"They may make it possible to tell whether the treatment has eradicated the Lyme disease bacteria. And they therefore also make it possible to tell if a patient with a prior infection now has a new infection."[13]

---

12 "Lyme Disease Facts and Statistics," https://www.bayarealyme.org/ (Bay Area Lyme Foundation, July 21, 2022), https://www.bayarealyme.org/about-lyme/lyme-disease-facts-statistics/.

13 Julie Rafferty, "A Potential New Test for Diagnosing Lyme Disease," https://now.tufts.edu/ (Tufts Now, March 15, 2022), https://now.tufts.edu/2022/03/15/potential-new-test-diagnosing-lyme-disease.

So *fast-forward*, Brian had a challenging high school experience, but he made it through college. And today he's an engineer doing great for himself. But it's taken him from 2009 until now to get his life back together. One thing we know: the longer Lyme disease goes undiagnosed, the more dangerous it becomes.

Dr. Tennant teaches us that our bodies need the right tools to rebuild and restore, and if you're providing it voltage, detox, and nutrition, then restoration can happen. Dr. Jerry Tennant's confident work can change the paradigm of Western medicine. These FDA-accepted, noninvasive therapies offer healthcare professionals and home users affordable, drug-free, and user-friendly options for the indicated use of symptomatic relief for chronic, severe, and intractable pain, as well as treatment in the management of post-surgical and post-traumatic pain.

My practice of biologic dentistry has changed the way I do "history and physical." I look at what meds my patients take and ask them why. I know what supplements they use, especially if they have fatigue. A lot of people come in mentally tired. They've had their thyroid checked. They've had the physician clear them. Their blood work seems fine. *But why do they feel like crap?*

And I question.

I question traditional *everything*: traditional medicine, traditional dentistry. Not that I'm skeptical, but I've been exposed to a lot of things that I know potentially can work. (To be completely honest, I take a bit of mischievous delight in questioning the status quo.)

And if it is not working, you must make sure you go back to your primary physician, or your pediatrician, making sure that your child gets the best care and does not slip back, making measurable progress. And all my children have been in forward progress based on probiotics, nutrition, supplementation, exercise programs, physical therapy, and energy medicine.

I had another patient with a tough foot issue, a toe issue that very talented physicians just could not figure out. I traced through the meridians. I shared the meridian chart with the patient. We identified the tooth that the meridian chart indicated would be a direction to look for a dental issue. We did that. And after we took the 3D x-ray cone beam CT scan, the physician and patient decided that it might be best to remove the tooth and the infection surrounding it, and the toe infection cleared up right away.

But because of that, I'm saying to myself, *You know what? We don't deal with just teeth. We deal with how teeth affect parts of the body and how the corresponding parts of the body affect teeth.*

Every tooth that has a problem could be sending out a message. It can be an organ problem or a glandular problem, affecting the tooth along one of the twelve *meridians*, a system that I've gained great confidence in using as a diagnostic guide.

The easy solution may not be the right solution. *Oh, my tooth hurts … take it out or do a root canal on it … or do a filling on it*—but that may not be the primary source of the problem.

In my next chapter, we'll explore the meridian chart and how it came to be such a powerful diagnostic tool to help associate a tooth with an organ based on an individual's medical history. Chinese medicine scholars discovered the energy meridians over five thousand years ago. Commonly known as acupuncture meridians, or acupressure points, several medical disciplines consider them.

Often chided as being like astral charts, meridians are invisible highways in the body that are grounded in centuries of Chinese medicine, and they can guide a diagnostic inquiry very accurately. There are those flat earthers who flinch when a clinician mentions meridians. They abide by the one-answer-that-rules-them-all temper of our times. I try to be a prudent steward of this ancient wisdom and apply the theory as a guide in diagnostics. I got out of my defensive crouch years ago. This stuff works, and it gets very interesting.

You will enjoy the next chapter. Truth carries its own light.

DENTAL MERIDIANS, ANCIENT WISDOM, AND DIAGNOSTIC WAYFINDING TO BETTER HEALTH

It seems like yesterday, but in the summer of 2007, Jay W. Friedman, DDS, MPH published an article in the *American Journal of Public Health* that turned the common practice of wisdom teeth removal on its ear. Dr. Friedman has devoted his career to championing evidence-based dental care.

His article offered the headline, "The Prophylactic Extraction of Third Molars: A Public Health Hazard." And he meant it.

Dr. Friedman reminded us that (as of 2007) ten million third molars (wisdom teeth) were extracted from approximately five million people in the United States each year at an annual cost of over $3 billion.

In addition, he offered the math that "more than eleven million patient days of "standard discomfort or disability"—pain, swelling, bruising, and malaise—result postoperatively, and more than eleven thousand people suffer permanent paresthesia—numbness of the lip, tongue, and cheek—as a consequence of nerve injury during the surgery."

At least two-thirds of these extractions, he offered, resulted in unnecessary costs and injuries, "constituting a silent epidemic of iatrogenic (relating to illness caused by medical examination or treatment) injury that afflicts tens of thousands of people with lifelong discomfort and disability."[14]

Dr. Friedman cited data that not more than 12 percent of impacted teeth have associated pathology (*a clinical reason for removal*). He notes the same incidence for appendicitis (10 percent) and cholecystitis (12 percent), yet prophylactic (*medicine or course of action used to prevent disease*) appendectomies and cholecystectomies are not the standards of care.

And he asks the dental profession, "Why then prophylactic third-molar extractions?"

Well, that sealed the deal for me. I had never advocated the removal of uncomplicated wisdom teeth. I agreed with Dr. Friedman. It meets the definition of public health hazard.

---

14   J. W. Friedman, "The Prophylactic Extraction of Third Molars: A Public Health Hazard," *American Journal of Public Health*, https://www.ncbi.nlm.nih.gov/pmc/articles/PMC1963310/.

CHAPTER 2

Truth Carries Its Own Light

I mention wisdom teeth as an introduction to dental meridians. Not only does this subject fall into the conservative, "first do no harm" minimally invasive mantra of holistic dentistry, but it clearly illustrates the fact that our teeth should not be viewed as something apart from the rest of our body. Teeth connect to every single cell, to every single organ in our body, and therefore are intimately correlated to our bodily functions, organ systems, tissues, and cellular health.

We are a single miraculous organism with everything entirely interconnected and interdependent. We human beings have a wonderful design: a fluid, dynamic, and permeable biology.

So almost everybody gets their wisdom teeth extracted anywhere from age eighteen to twenty-five, right? Let's say in the United States, 60 percent of us do. (I have seen estimates up to 90 percent.)

I always ask my patients if they have ever had a dry socket from an extraction, especially a wisdom tooth. If you have four pulled or cut out all at once, and you are eighteen, and you go jogging the next day or do something silly like that, you can very quickly develop an infection in one of those spaces, and the body will not heal properly. Those spaces may develop into what we call an *osteonecrotic lesion*, a potential source of chronic, long-term infection. Each of our teeth associates with an organ of the body. Our wisdom teeth, particularly the wisdom teeth sites number one, number sixteen, number seventeen, and number thirty-two, are associated with the heart through the meridians.

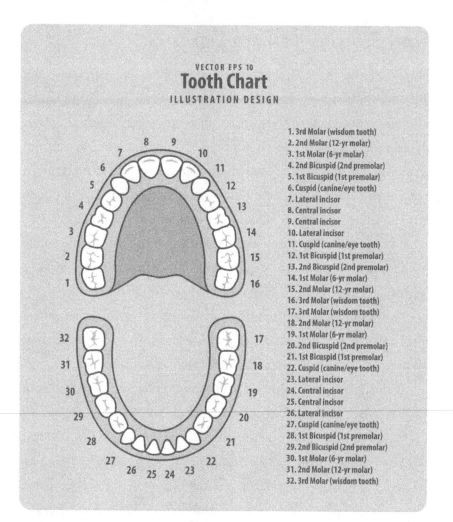

So, how many people develop major heart issues in their sixties? I believe, based on experience and training, that your risk of heart issues could involve wisdom teeth. Holistic dentists already know this because we have seen the direct impact on problematic dental issues and whole-body health. The twelve meridians offer wayfinding, a road map, and a cue to go check out the part of the body joined to a problematic tooth by a meridian. One day, the data will likely support our belief in a direct connection between proactive wisdom tooth extraction and heart problems later in life.

The Chinese understood that energy flows within the body and affects our health and well-being, and specifically, regulates our organs. In the same way that arteries carry blood, meridians carry energy, often referred to as Qi (pronounced "chee") in Eastern medicine. Energy meridians are also strong influencers of immune system health and are often studied by functional medical doctors and naturopathic physicians in individuals with autoimmune disorders or flawed immune responses.

Over five millennia of practice, traditional Chinese medicine or "TCM" allowed the doctors to determine various disturbances in the flow of Qi energy along the meridians, which helps physicians understand the disease, illness, and abnormalities within patterns of cellular organization and growth. We have a tough time getting our arms around the five thousand years of development. Five thousand years ago, our Western culture was not developing such medicine. We were still centuries away from discovering the wheel, quietly painting beautiful murals on canyon walls.

Energy flows and energy meridians are invisible to the naked eye and imperceptible to all but the most trained medical practitioners like energy workers, kinesiologists, and holistic dentists. Centuries ago, traditional Chinese medicine practitioners could diagnose patients by tracking these subtle energies as they flow through the pathways of the human body or our energy meridians.

But when you go back to the basis of the meridians we use today, it is based on eons of Chinese medicine. They figured out which pathways are connected energetically and where they trace through the body. And centuries later, they discovered acupuncture points. Then, these two disciplines, meridians and acupuncture, came together. Being an electrical engineer, I visualize them as electrical bundles.

BIOLOGICAL RHYTHMS

Despite the absence of the term *biological rhythm*, traditional Chinese medicine (TCM) theory embraces the rhythmic phenomenon of the human being, such as circadian rhythm (daily rhythm) that has been studied most, as well as syzygial rhythm (lunar rhythm) and seasonal rhythm (annual rhythm).[15]

While energy flows and energy meridians are invisible to the naked eye and practically imperceptible to all but the most trained medical practitioners like kinesiologists and holistic dentists, centuries ago, the Chinese traditional medicine practitioners were able to diagnose patients by tracking this subtle energy as it flows through the pathways of the human body or our energy meridians.

The function of Qi and blood circulation represents the basic features of human vitality and the intrinsic connections among Yin and Yang, the five elements, viscera, Qi and blood, and other traditional Chinese medicine theories, thereby having a profound influence on the overall theoretical construction of traditional Chinese medicine.

Acupuncture and its various forms have evolved over the last two to three thousand years. The concepts of meridians and acupoints along meridians originated empirically as practitioners sought to understand and explain the sensations evoked during stimulation that appeared to radiate down lines along extremities and the body torso.

---

15   "Tianxing Zhang et al., "Human Biological Rhythm in Traditional Chinese Medicine," https://www.sciencedirect.com/ (*Journal of Traditional Chinese Medical Sciences*, October 2016), https://www.sciencedirect.com/science/article/pii/S2095754816301028.

Today, I encourage traditional acupuncture and also use a dental laser (it's kind of a needleless acupuncture). My patients with headaches benefit from acupuncture.

I have a strong belief in the use of acupuncture. Years ago, when I hyperextended my elbow, I knew the value of acupuncture to establish a blood flow to the area to increase healing. I also use this therapy for upper shoulder issues. I have knots in the trapezius areas that give me wicked headaches. The acupuncturist does a one-needle acupuncture placement that reduces pain and inflammation and relieves the headache. My son Luke has also used acupuncture for general wellness and to help with other issues.

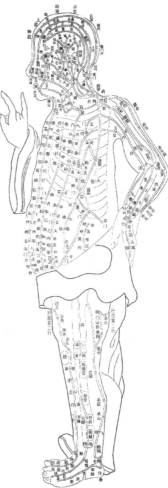

I have a patient with painful trigeminal neuralgia that I send to a Chinese acupuncturist. One might assume that the acupuncture would be happening on the face, but she places needles in different parts of his body, the acupuncture areas, the meridians that establish a Qi, or a flow of energy, to try to reduce inflammation in the zone, which improves the outcome.

Over fifty accredited schools of acupuncture reside in the United States. If you wish to find an acupuncture practitioner, there should be one relatively close to home.

The Flow of Rivers

Early medicine in China involved the symbolic analogy of the flow of rivers and the irrigation system of agriculture. The meridian theory "is abstract and yet concrete, dialectic and yet intuitive, definite and yet vague, integrated and yet independent, having a profound influence on the overall formation of traditional Chinese medicine theories."[16]

Thousands of years ago, the people of China, an agricultural society, deeply felt that the condition of an irrigation system determines the harvest. "The flow of water over streams and mountains is a natural phenomenon and part of the natural environment; it is also closely related to agricultural production. As the way of human beings resembles that of heaven, the human body will certainly have a system of Qi and blood circulation similar to that of rivers and lakes in nature."[17]

Scholars still debate the exact time of birth for the meridian concept. Archaeologists did find a brief description of the eleven meridians in the silk manuscripts excavated from Mawangdui Han Tombs. Still, later, the meridian theory had matured in its development around the time of the Yellow Emperor's Canon of Medicine. *The Canon* (2600 BC) has made it clear that as the earth has four seas in the east, south, west, and north, the human body must also have four "seas," namely, the sea of Shuigu (food digestion), the sea of Twelve Meridians, the sea of Qi, and the sea of Marrow, and as there are twelve rivers on earth, so there must be twelve meridians inside the human body.

---

16   Li Lei, Ching Wo Tung, and Kwai Ching Lo, "The Origin of Meridians," scirp.org (Scientific Research Publishing, May 2, 2014), https://www.scirp.org/html/3-8801198_46074.htm.

17   Ibid.

It also established the basic framework of the twelve meridian system,[18] depicting meridians as an inter-connected system of circulation. This ancient Chinese medical text has been treated as the fundamental doctrinal source for Chinese medicine for more than two millennia and until today. Many compare it in importance to the *Hippocratic Corpus* in Greek medicine or the works of Galen in Islamic and medieval European medicine.

A meridian does not describe an anatomical structure. Its morphology has not been in any way traced inside the human body. We have learned that theories of traditional Chinese medicine are constructed mainly upon the basis of philosophical thinking, emphasizing a broad understanding of the body's functional status as a whole, making the anatomical description of human structures less important or even dispensable. The meridian theory has apparently reflected the perceptual characteristics of Chinese culture for its direct image visualization with intuitive logic, which must be a key point when we discuss the origin of meridians.

The twelve meridians are like superhighways. Research on these acupuncture meridians found an 80 percent correspondence between the sites of acupuncture points and the location of connected tissue planes in postmortem tissue specimens. For the first time, scientists could see that meridians are not just theory, and they said, *Do you know what? There's validity to this.*

More recently, practitioners have tried to identify anatomical structures that represent meridians "but, as of yet, according to the *Journal of Acupuncture and Meridian Studies*, structures such as tendinomuscular meridians and primo-vessels (Bonghan ducts) have

---

18   Li Zhaoguo, Liu Xiru, *The Yellow Emperor's Canon of Medicine, Plain Conversation*, Library of Chinese Classics English & Chinese Edition 2004, May 1, 2004.

not been shown to serve physiologically or clinically as meridians as originally proposed by early practitioners."[19]

The importance lies in how caregivers use the ancient wisdom of meridians.

A patient who seeks care from the dentist reports that *I have a toothache*. Okay. Let's look. We hope we will find just that, a tooth problem. But then we trace the meridian to the tooth involved. Biologic dentistry will take the tooth problem as a cue to look at the whole body. The tooth no doubt has a problem, but that's not necessarily the source of the problem. The problem could be in the lungs, intestines, liver, or gallbladder, and it shows up in your mouth as a tooth issue. This wayfinding represents the essence of the value of the meridian chart. The science of the twelve meridians provides a cue to check it out. In working with the tooth, we trace it back and ask the patient, *Do you have any issues in these areas highlighted by the meridian for this tooth?*

It can work both ways. The meridian serves as a two-way street. You can have a tooth that affects an organ or an organ that affects the tooth. Now, of course, I do not diagnose organ issues or glandular issues. I'll state something like, *I cannot see why this tooth bothers you. We can treat you for the pain, give it some time, and see if the issue heals, or I can send you back to your physician, and you can ask questions about, let's say, your liver, kidney, or thyroid.* That's how I pragmatically use meridian lines.

Most physicians leave dental or oral issues to the dentist to find the problem because they're not schooled in it. Then it's pretty straightforward. The 3D x-rays are very detailed today, showing if there's a cavity, an abscess (developing abscess), or an undetected bone lesion.

---

19   John C. Longhurst, "Defining Meridians: A Modern Basis of Understanding," *Journal of Acupuncture and Meridian Studies* 3, no. 2 (June 2010): 67–74, https://www.sciencedirect.com/journal/journal-of-acupuncture-and-Meridian-studies.

Many doctors understand that problems in the mouth can affect the whole body, so maybe that is why the patient does not feel well. Many smart doctors will send their patients to a biologic dentist to evaluate the mouth and rule out the absence of dental disease.

And if the physician can cross that off the equation, then the physician has a better chance of solving the problem. Dentists do not diagnose issues below the collarbone, but we suggest an examination of the patient with an eye on specific areas of the body as announced by the painful tooth and its meridian. *Hey, it would be best if you discussed with your physician that you might have a problem with your gallbladder.* Because, potentially, this tooth that's showing up as a "nonissue" traces back to your gallbladder.

So, we deeply value a back-and-forth dentist-doctor relationship. The tooth could be compared to a circuit breaker. You should have energy running freely through your twelve meridians. If a tooth causes a portion of the problem or has become the problem, it can slow down or act as an electrical drain on that meridian or that organ. Our body needs the proper voltage for our cells and the proper voltage to perform correctly. And if it drops below a certain level, you can start developing a disease. The body needs steady energy to run efficiently. It has to find this energy from other areas to keep the cells working optimally or functionally. It can become more of a drain on the system in that meridian or an adjacent meridian.

Dr. Jerry Tennant writes about this subject and how bacteria flow from a tooth through the meridians.

"If you have decay in a tooth and you're trying to put a circuit through there, you can see how the decay would act as a resistor and drop the voltage. In addition, if you have an infection from a tooth that goes out into the bone around it, which always happens in a root canal tooth (because the tooth has died), eventually, the infection passes from the tooth into the bone around it. As it passes into the bone, it shorts the circuit out almost completely, and that can cause the polarity to flip."

Dr. Tennant also notes that you can have the same happen if you had a tooth pulled and acquired an infection in the bone. Again, he frequently finds a common problem with people developing any illness: an infection in a bone around a tooth.

"By the way, that infection can be there for thirty or forty years and not cause pain but then short the circuit out," he adds.[20]

Dr. Tennant teaches that bacterial infections in a tooth produce particles almost indistinguishable from viruses. These are very destructive toxins. "They pass along the associated acupuncture meridian causing damage to everything wired to that meridian." For example, an infection in any one of the teeth associated with the eye can cause uvulitis. I view it as my responsibility to pay close attention to my patients with root canals. We must make sure that any organ trouble, or non-tooth trouble, is not related. A tooth in that meridian could well be a cause (or potential cause) of that organ issue, Dr. Tennant notes.[21]

Dr. Jerry Tennant makes sure that 100 percent of his patients do not have dental infections, which could be causing a problem with an organ. For instance, my wife Susan struggled with dry eyes, ocular inflammation. He first made sure that she had a dental exam with a 3D x-ray to make sure that a tooth did not cause her eye issue. And how would that be? That tooth might be preventing that meridian system from operating efficiently. I did the 3D x-ray on her and an oral exam. In her case, it was not.

Well, there are physicians, the naturopath, and nurse practitioners in the holistic field that send patients to me for assessment, to make

---

20   The Tennant Institute for Integrative Medicine, "A Detailed Look at the 5 Factors of Low Voltage," accessed August 22, 2022, https://tennantinstitute.com/5-factors-of-low-voltage/.

21   Ibid.

sure that dentally they are cleared, because an issue, a systemic issue, can come from several areas. And they want to rule out the dental connection, and they want a biologic dentist who knows how to do that.

So, we screen for blood pressure because people come to the dentist more often than their primary care provider. The American Dental Association requests that we do blood pressure checks on our patients annually. When we find elevated blood pressure, we wind up sending them back to their physician, and we often hear back, *Wow, oh wow. Your dentist gets a gold star today*! We also ask if the patient sleeps well.

French diplomat George Soulié de Morant brought acupuncture to Europe in the early 1900s after serving in China. He coined the terms *meridian* and *energy*. With the founding of a new China in 1949, Western medicine in the region also began to play a large role in medical care. As Westernized medicine's impact increased, "integrative medicine" evolved at the end of the 1950s. Theories, therapeutic principles, technologies, and understanding of the life sciences were elaborated, and the basic structure of traditional Chinese medicine also became better understood.

Biologic dentistry embraces these invisible pathways. We have seen the connections every day for years. I can be a conservative, pragmatic dentist and have a profound belief in the meridian theory because I am certain it can help my patients to better health.

Our next chapter on the explicit, visible hazard of heavy metals in the mouth is not based on such ancient science, centuries of devotion, and intuitive knowledge. It's based on historical amnesia, debates over time, recent dental history, and modern environmental science. They called this the *amalgam wars*. And it got ugly. What you cannot see can hurt you.

HEAVY METALS AND "THE MAD HATTER": WHAT YOU CANNOT SEE CAN HURT YOU

A land was full of wonder, mystery, and danger. Some say to survive it, you need to be as mad as a hatter. Which, luckily, I am.[22]

Alice in Wonderland

—LEWIS CARROLL, 1865

Author Lewis Carroll did not coin the term "mad hatter," noted the celebrated medical writer Laura Lane in her 2007 two-part historical series on mercury amalgam.

"It entered the late 18th century to mid-19th centuries when hat factory workers often babbled nonsense and behaved irrationally," she described. "These signs, along with tremors, psychosis, and hallucinations, stemmed from inhaling vapors of mercury, which helped soften material used for making hats."[23]

---

22   Lewis Carroll and Sir John Tenniel, *Alice's Adventures in Wonderland* (New York: Macmillan, November 1865).

23   Laura Lane, "Amalgam Wars: Part I—A Phantom Menace?" Drbicuspid.com, accessed September 3, 2022, https://www.drbicuspid.com/index.aspx?sec=ser&sub=def&pag=dis&ItemID=300238.

Laura Lane also noted that dentists of that period may have risked similar symptoms when they mixed their own amalgam for fillings. "The process involved measuring the correct amount of mercury and using a mortar and pestle to blend in powdered metallic alloy," said Karl-Johan Söderholm, DDS, PhD, professor of materials science and engineering at the University of Florida.

This chapter aims to alert you to the prospect of a health threat and to give you the tools to self-assess what's in your mouth. Like all my biologic dentistry practices, the choice will be up to you. This is the behind-the-scenes story of mercury and a fascinating tale.

As an engineer and a doctor, I know that elemental mercury represents a significant danger. Many of us came to that conclusion and became mercury-free and mercury safe, deciding not to place amalgams in patients anymore. Internationally, agreements have just emerged to cease mercury fillings in young children and pregnant women.

I know some recent dental school graduates in America have never placed one amalgam filling, and I celebrate that. They have refused to add to the mercury burden that is already existing and have embraced the training on becoming mercury-safe practitioners.

The International Academy of Oral Medicine and Toxicology (IAOMT), concerned about mercury exposure, seeks to eliminate the dangers.

"The process of drilling out amalgam fillings liberates quantities of mercury vapor and fine particulates that can be inhaled and absorbed through the lungs, potentially harmful to patients, dentists, dental workers, and their fetuses." (In fact, the IAOMT does not recommend that pregnant women have their amalgams removed.)

Based on up-to-date scientific research, the IAOMT developed rigorous recommendations for removing existing dental mercury amalgam fillings to reduce the potential adverse health outcomes of mercury exposure to patients, dental professionals, dental students, office staff, and others. The IAOMT created the Safe Mercury Amalgam Removal Technique (SMART).

SMART exists for all dentists who want to expand safety protocols for themselves, their staff, and their patients. It reduces the amount of mercury being redistributed from the existing filling into the room and into the air that the practitioner and the assistants breathe. And, even more importantly, into the patient, where they reabsorb it in another form, which is also being aerosolized while vaporized. Patients breathe that, and they swallow it. SMART trains us to acquire safety equipment and use barrier techniques, pre-rinses, and supplemental air to benefit the patient, the staff, the dentist, and our environment.

A Phantom Menace

Laura Lane's 2007 historical treatise on amalgam represents one of the most revealing histories of this controversy. She had cut her teeth for years spent in medical journalism. She first sank her incisors into newspapers and then moved on to the molar-grinding dot-com world. She has written for the *Dallas Morning News, Harvard Women's Health Letter, Shape* magazine, and WebMD. She earned a BS in biology from the University of California, Los Angeles, and an MS in biological sciences from Stanford University.[24]

Laura Lane published her treatise on the DrBicuspid website. DrBicuspid.com provides a free, member-driven website dedicated to general dentists, specialists, and other dental professionals to deliver practical, trustworthy, relevant news, features, columns, and more that will help practicing dentists.

---

24   Ibid.

Lane called the amalgam controversy a "phantom menace" in that powerful two-part series on the history of the use of mercury in dentistry.[25]

"Like the monster in some Grade B horror flick, the argument over amalgam fillings just will not die," she wrote. The argument in America began well before the War Between the States.

Every year, Lane noted, a scientist steps forward, brandishing the results of a new study designed to drive a stake through its heart. "But before the journal leaves the printing press, opposing scientists pick it apart. What makes this question so hard to answer?"

In 2007, she alerted the world that mercury, one of the most toxic substances on the planet, has been a problem for nearly two centuries and that desperate warnings have been sounded to stop the use of (low-cost) amalgam fillings to repair our teeth.

The use of silver amalgam in dentistry dates back to seventh-century China. Still, the material didn't find its way into Westerners' teeth until the nineteenth century, according to the 1998 book *The Excruciating History of Dentistry: Toothsome Tales & Oral Oddities from Babylon to Braces.* By then, mercury's toxic properties were well known, and amalgam fillings swiftly became controversial on both sides of the Atlantic.[26]

Few people dispute that chewing on amalgam fillings releases mercury vapor or that some of the vapor finds its way into the lungs. Few argue that mercury can cause damage. From the lungs, mercury vapor passes into red blood cells, oxidizing them, becoming mercuric ion. Mercuric ion tends to accumulate in the brain and kidneys, which bind to sulfur in essential proteins, denying them to cells. Deprived of these proteins, cells die. While the body eventually eliminates some mercury, a portion remains sequestered in these organs.

---

25 Ibid.

26 James Wybrandt, *The Excruciating History of Dentistry: Toothsome Tales & Oral Oddities from Babylon to Braces* (New York: St. Martin's Griffin, 2000).

TWO CENTURIES OF NASTY DEBATE

1833

Englishman Edward Crawcour and his nephew Moses Crawcour opened a dental practice in New York in 1833, where they used the "new" amalgam of silver and mercurial, the so-called silver fillings. The fillings were supposed to replace gold, which was then the standard filler material and also much cheaper. After a few years, amalgam was declared an extremely bad tooth-filling material that also caused sickly changes in the mouth and all sorts of terrible side effects.[27]

1835

American dentists organized into groups that forbade members to use amalgam. However, amalgam's advantages were far too significant for dentists to pass up. Because it was much cheaper, dentists could extend their services beyond those wealthy enough to afford the precious metal and easier to work with and more malleable than gold.

1843: The First Amalgam War

The American Society of Dental Surgeons (ASDS), founded in New York, declared the use of amalgam to be malpractice because of the fear of mercury poisoning in patients and dentists and forced all its members to sign a pledge to abstain from using it, initiating the beginning of the controversy.[28]

1848

The debate became so divisive that it has been dubbed the *amalgam wars.*[29] Many American Dental Association members were excommunicated. In 1848, eleven dentists were excluded from the Dental Association in New York because they had neglected their patients by using amalgam.

---

27   Ibid.

28   Monika Rathore, Archana Singh, and Vandana A. Pant, "The Dental Amalgam Toxicity Fear: A Myth or Actuality," National Library of Medicine, accessed September 5, 2022, https://www.ncbi.nlm.nih.gov/pmc/articles/PMC3388771/.

29   Monika Rathore, Archana Singh, and Vandana A Pant, "The Dental Amalgam Toxicity Fear: A Myth or Actuality," https://www.ncbi.nlm.nih.gov/ (U.S. National Library of Medicine, May 2012), https://www.ncbi.nlm.nih.gov/pmc/articles/PMC3388771/.

1895

With experimentation, the material evolved. Dentists added tin to the silver-mercury mix, which prevented fillings from expanding in the patients' teeth. By 1895, the formula was more or less standardized: 50 percent mercury, 35 percent silver, 9 percent tin, 6 percent copper, and a trace of zinc. Membership in the American Society of Dental Surgeons, the leading anti-amalgam group, declined to the point that the organization disbanded in 1856. Three years later, the American Dental Association rose in its place. From the beginning, the new organization took a stand in favor of the controversial material.

1926: The Second Amalgam War

In 1926, German chemist Alfred Stock called out with his warnings about using mercurial amalgam. Stock published his experiences about mercurial poisoning, having become very ill from a slowly insidious mercurial poisoning. He described his symptoms in detail, which included mental disturbances, irregular heart activity, trembling, dizziness, depression, and other symptoms. He moved to a "Hg-free laboratory." (Today, the element mercury on the periodic table retains its Hg abbreviation—a nod to its old Latin name, hydrargyrum, which means "water silver.") Alfred Stock removed his mercurial fillings, replacing them with friendlier materials, and he recovered from his severe mercurial poisoning and contributed important findings to research.

Present day: The Third Amalgam War

The US has fallen behind other developed nations in confronting toxic mercury, and we still languish in the advanced stages of the third amalgam war. The argument was reopened in the late 1970s, as modern methods of detecting the presence of trace amounts of mercury were introduced, including mass spectrophotometry and the Jerome mercury vapor detector. Swedish neurobiologist Mats Hansen, reviewing a series of early and mid-twentieth-century studies, sent a letter to the Swedish National Board of Health demanding an unprejudiced evaluation of the hazards of dental mercury amalgam. Due to Hansen and others' efforts, Sweden banned the use of amalgams in pregnant women in 1987.

Although the cause of the anti-amalgamists in America renewed slowly in the mid-1980s, it gained momentum in the 1990s.

Source: Laura Lane

A Nutty Idea

The Journal of the American Medical Association (JAMA) published two randomized, prospective clinical trials carefully aimed at detecting a health threat connected to mercury content in dental fillings. They found no cause for concern.[30]

Lane notes in her amalgam wars history that David Bellinger, PhD, MSc, an author of one of the JAMA studies, can understand why the public, and some dentists, remain confused. "It does seem like a nutty idea to put a heavy metal in your mouth," said Dr. Bellinger, a professor of environmental health at the Harvard School of Public Health.[31] Lane reminds us that the "seemingly nutty idea" dates back hundreds of years. No other metal exists as a liquid at room temperature, a property that earned the element the nickname "quicksilver." This attribute also accounts for its popularity among early metal workers; it can easily combine with other metals to form amalgams. In nature, mercury chemically ties to sulfur, where it does no harm. Once workers release it from these bonds, the metal can kill.

In the air, elemental mercury vapor passes through the lungs into the bloodstream. In water, microorganisms convert elemental mercury to methylmercury. This compound, found in fish, can pass through the gastrointestinal tract into the bloodstream. Worldwide, scientists

---

30 David C. Bellinger, Felicia Trachtenberg, Lars Barregard, Mary Tavares, Elsa Cernichiari, David Daniel, and Sonja McKinlay, "Neuropsychological and Renal Effects of Dental Amalgam in Children: A Randomized Clinical Trial," *Journal of the American Medical Association* (April 19, 2006).

31 Laura Lane, "Amalgam Wars: Part II—A Phantom Menace?," Drbicuspid.com, accessed September 3, 2022, https://www.drbicuspid.com/index.aspx?sec=ser&sub=def&pag=dis&ItemID=300248.

have agreed that through either route, mercury can enter and damage other organs, including the brain.

A significant example of mercury exposure affecting public health occurred in Minamata, Japan, between 1932 and 1968, where a factory producing acetic acid discharged waste liquid into Minamata Bay. The discharge included high concentrations of methylmercury. The bay was rich in fish and shellfish, providing the main livelihood for local residents and fishermen from other areas. For years, no one realized that the fish were contaminated with mercury and that it was causing a strange disease in the local community and other districts. At least fifty thousand people were affected to some extent, and more than two thousand cases of Minamata disease were certified. Minamata disease peaked in the 1950s, with severe cases suffering brain damage, paralysis, incoherent speech, and delirium.[32]

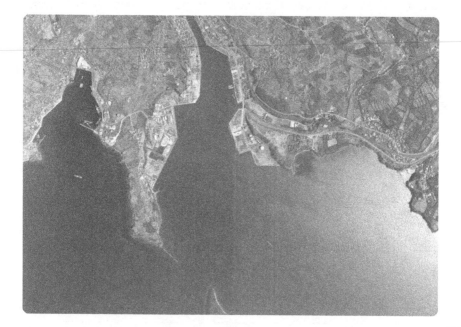

---

32   World Health Organization, "Mercury and Health," https://www.who.int/news-room/fact-sheets/
      detail/mercury-and-health#:~:text=Mercury%20may%20have%20toxic%20effects,of%20major%20
      public%20health%20concern, March 31, 2017.

The international agreements surrounding the issue of mercury pollution have been negotiated by The Minamata Convention, named as such in memory of the Japanese disaster. The group works together to create global treaties to protect human health and the environment from the adverse effects of mercury.

In the invitation to attend these conferences, the leadership lays it out:

"Considerable scientific knowledge has been developed on sources and emissions of mercury, its fate, pathways and cycling through the environment, human exposure, and effects on human health. An agreement has been reached among scientists that mercury exposure today threatens human health. This scientific knowledge, obtained through studies conducted in various research centers on all continents, formed the basis for policymakers' decision to establish an international agreement on the reduction of emissions and exposure to mercury."[33]

Charlie Brown, the executive director of Consumers for Dental Choice, has evolved into a major champion for this campaign for mercury-free dentistry. Brown led more than forty organizations representing children, the environment, ethics, consumers, and health professionals to advocate for filling the vacancy of Chief Dental Officer of the Public Health Service. They wanted a new leader who will immediately stop the use of mercury dental fillings in children and pregnant women—then phase out its use entirely in federal programs. He created quite a squabble.

Europe leads the United States in reducing that, with recent steps to protect children under fifteen, pregnant women, and breastfeeding mothers from amalgams at the Minamata Convention on Mercury. (The US is a signatory.) The World Health Organization now favors minimally invasive, mercury-free dentistry.

---

33   "We Are Pleased to Welcome You to ICMGP 2019 in Krakow!," https://mercury2019krakow.com/gb/ (International Conference on Mercury as a Global Pollutant, 2019), https://mercury2019krakow.com/gb/information.html.

THE TEN CHEMICALS OF PUBLIC HEALTH CONCERN[34]

1. Air pollution
2. Arsenic
3. Asbestos
4. Benzene
5. Cadmium
6. Dioxins and dioxin-like substances
7. Inadequate or excess fluoride
8. Lead
9. Mercury
10. Highly hazardous pesticides

David Brooks, prolific columnist for the *New York Times*, wrote in a 2013 essay that "life is a partnership among the dead, the living, and the unborn, with obligations to those to come."[35]

According to the WHO, the unborn are the most susceptible to developmental effects due to mercury. Methylmercury exposure in the womb can result from a mother's consumption of fish and shellfish. It can adversely affect a baby's growing brain and nervous system. Scientists believe that the primary health effect of methylmercury manifests as impaired neurological development. Therefore, cognitive thinking, memory, attention, language, and fine motor and visual-spatial skills may be affected in children who were exposed to methylmercury as fetuses.

People regularly exposed to high levels of mercury, such as populations that rely on subsistence fishing or people occupationally exposed, face an imminent threat to their health. Among selected subsistence fishing populations, between 1.5 out of 1,000 and 17 out of 1,000 children showed cognitive impairment (mild mental

---

34 World Health Organization (WHO), "Mercury and Health," March 31, 2017.

35 David Brooks, "Carpe Diem Nation," *New York Times*, February 11, 2013, https://www.nytimes.com/2013/02/12/opinion/brooks-carpe-diem-nation.html.

retardation) caused by the consumption of fish containing mercury. These included populations in Brazil, Canada, China, Columbia, and Greenland.[36]

The WHO notes that neurological and behavioral disorders may be observed after inhalation, ingestion, or dermal exposure of different mercury compounds. Symptoms include tremors, insomnia, memory loss, neuromuscular effects, headaches, and cognitive and motor dysfunction.

THE CLEVELAND CLINIC

Elemental Mercury Poisoning Symptoms[37]

Elemental mercury is usually harmless if you touch or swallow it because its slippery texture won't absorb into your skin or intestines. Elemental mercury is extremely dangerous if you breathe it in and it gets into your lungs. Often, elemental mercury becomes airborne if someone is trying to clean up a mercury spill with a vacuum.

Symptoms of elemental mercury poisoning occur immediately after inhaling the chemical and include:

- Coughing
- Trouble breathing
- Metallic taste in your mouth
- Nausea or vomiting
- Bleeding or swollen gums

Inorganic Mercury Poisoning Symptoms

Inorganic mercury is poisonous when swallowed. When the chemical enters your body, it travels through your bloodstream and attacks your brain and kidneys.

---

36   "Mercury and Health," who.int (World Health Organization, March 31, 2017), https://www.who.int/news-room/fact-sheets/detail/mercury-and-health.

37   "Mercury Poisoning: Symptoms, Causes & Treatment," https://my.clevelandclinic.org/ (Cleveland Clinic, 2022), https://my.clevelandclinic.org/health/diseases/23420-mercury-poisoning.

Symptoms of inorganic mercury poisoning include:

- Burning sensation in your stomach and/or throat
- Nausea or vomiting
- Diarrhea
- Blood in vomit or stool

It is a win-win-win that we protect everybody when removing amalgam.

"... Before Our Awakening"

Being a mercury-safe dentist, I use the protocols to remove it in a safer way than we did years ago, before our awakening. We invest in the process. We store the mercury materials in a separate container, usually filled with a liquid or water, so it does not release gas. A special carrier picks that up with a chain of custody and all the signatures and the protocol. We know it is responsibly handled.

Not cheap, but it's really cheap to put in that filling in the first place. It does offer a cheaper filling, but that "cheap" creates a great expense in the long run, potentially damaging to the health of everyone involved and the environment.

I leased a mercury sniffer (mercury vapor detector) to test inside my operatory, and because of our discipline and caution, it barely registered anything, well under the EPA standard for a hazard area.

In the 1980s and 1990s, they would offer testing at large dental meetings. They tested the blood to check for mercury issues. But they were testing for acute heavy metal toxicity through a blood test, not ideal. The body absorbs mercury, first of all, intracellularly. If you are using a blood test, you may not find it because it has already been absorbed within the cell. If you get a "heavy metal test," you must tease the metals out with a chelation challenge test or use a very specific lab like the mercury tri-test to see what your mercury burden really looks like.

I believe dentists, in the past, before glove days, were being exposed to mercury. Created in the office, amalgam preparation started with a few metals, then wetted with mercury, squeezed with a cheesecloth, and finally, the dentist put the wetted amalgam into the tooth. That toxic mix was invisibly creating gases and potentially causing many people problems.

Then, amalgam evolved into using capsules, which had titrated mercury in one section. After you puncture it, it wets the metal, and you then place it in a triturator, which spins the material capsule at high RPMs to allow centrifugal force to mix the material evenly and smoothly. Then, you take that mercury and put it into the tooth through a carrier method.

Dr. Chris Slade has devoted his career to better testing and detoxification for mercury burdens to get a much clearer view, as well as other heavy metal toxins.

"Some of these toxins have an effect which is epigenetic or transgenerational where they will actually turn down the response systems (of future generations)," Dr. Chris Slade notes.

"This is one of the biggest areas where we need to look at mercury, as a community toxin—as something … affecting the whole gene pool," he adds.[38]

You can have all kinds of problems from the distribution of mercury throughout your body. You could have stomach problems or kidney problems. There is a high affinity for mercury in the kidney, and in the brain. You can have lung issues and digestive problems.

---

38   Chris Slade, "Quantifying Your Mercury Burden and Detoxification," The Quantified Body, accessed September 5, 2022, https://thequantifiedbody.net/quantifying-your-mercury-burden-dr-chris-shade/.

What do we replace amalgam with in our dental work? We use either zirconium-based crowns and implants, porcelains, ceramics, and composites, which can have their own issues too, because they are a plastic, and we still remain concerned because of that chemical composition. But it most certainly offers a practical alternative.

I wish to make a point here by including the chemical names of toxic materials that may be in composite materials. I do this to emphasize that these alternatives to mercury have been a scientifically based process, and the jury of experience is still out.

They selected mercury originally because it made hats softer and dental cement more pliable and easier to shape.

Composites may be toxic if they contain bisphenol A (BPA) or other toxic materials. As those fillings wear down over time, toxic materials used in the composite blend may seep into the body. Those materials include 2-hydroxyethyl methacrylate (HEMA) and bisphenol A-glycidyl methacrylate (bis-GMA), a bonding agent. Composite resins do vary, and most hold a variety of acrylics and other materials that allow for a bonding effect.

A biologic dentist using a whole-body approach will have already cleared this hurdle with you. Make sure your composite does not contain BPA and other potentially harmful materials. When doing the crowns or implants, we use materials more biocompatible, some less body-burdensome than others.

I guess we still have a standoff in the third amalgam war. It seems a pity that our culture calls every debate a *war*. We suffer from an undeniable strain of mercilessness. We certainly should not describe a clinical debate as a war. No practitioner should lose their license merely because they disagree with the opinion of the majority. The American Medical Association leaves these decisions to the dental community. But remember, dentistry has been using amalgams for almost two centuries. Amalgams clearly offer a lower-cost method to repair a tooth. It may take years for the evidence to stack up high enough to move the needle to mercury-free dentistry. In the meantime, more dentists have abandoned mercury fillings, as holistic and biologic dentistry practices gain in popularity.

I personally believe we have already passed a reasonable amount of time in debate, and the national oversight should

INVISIBLE HAZARDS ARE THE DEADLIEST.

insist on removing it from dentistry completely. Our culture finally did that with asbestos, but only after decades of pumping it into every building on earth. We should learn from the splinters and thorns of our history.

Invisible hazards are the deadliest.

In the absence of that long-overdue decision, dentists may tell their patients that it is their choice.

Even some highly regarded dentists still take the other side of this debate. A nice couple called recently to cancel their appointments. They called our office manager saying that they were having a really challenging time with their family because their son works as a dental hygienist, and his dentist said that "all this mercury stuff is bunk." The argument continues even within families.

I have a concern for hygienists who do not work in a mercury-free/mercury-safe practice. These fillings are thought to outgas through the life of the patient. When a hygienist polishes dental amalgams, they heat them up and use pumice. In heating, it creates a vapor. It's nice and shiny and does not collect plaque, because a rough surface would collect more plaque than a polished surface. This makes no sense to me, no sense at all.

Researchers agree that amalgam restorations leach mercury into the mouth, but a decision to fully address the threat has not yet happened.

It's invisible.

If we take amalgam fillings out in a safe clinical manner, everybody is protected. I do not see a reason we cannot take them out safely. If patients want them out, it is certainly their choice. The metallic color of amalgam does not blend with the natural tooth color, and consequently, both patients and professionals often prefer tooth-colored restorative material for cavity filling, for better aesthetics.[39]

IAOMT's SMART-certified members have completed a training course in the safe removal of dental mercury fillings. Accredited members have completed a comprehensive ten-unit course on biological dentistry, and masters and fellows have completed five hundred hours of additional research.

We have mercury testing available now, and I test my office often, something every dental practice should consider. Mercury does not just disappear over time.

SO MANY METALS

Louis Regnart, known as the "Father of Amalgam," improved on boiled mineral cement by adding mercury, which greatly reduced the high temperature originally needed to pour the cement onto a tooth. In the 1890s, G.V. Black gave a formula for dental amalgam that provided clinically acceptable performance and remained unchanged virtually for seventy years. In 1959, Dr. Wilmer Eames promoted low mercury-to-alloy mixing ratio. The mercury-to-amalgam ratio dropped from 8:5 to 1:1. The formula was again changed in 1963 when amalgam consisting of a high-copper dispersion alloy was introduced. It was later discovered

---

39   Ibid.

that the improved strength of the amalgam was a result of the additional copper forming a copper-tin phase that was less susceptible to corrosion than the tin-mercury phase in the earlier amalgam.[40]

Source: "The Dental Amalgam Toxicity Fear: A Myth or Actuality," National Library of Medicine

Dissimilar Metals

"You can have a battery already in your mouth and not even know it."

While the use of amalgam fillings placed by dentists in the United States has been declining, there still exist hundreds of millions of fillings, and these amalgam materials can react to other metals in the mouth. In 1979, the total number of amalgam restorations placed by dentists in the United States was estimated at 157,000,000.[41]

Now since that period, different formulas of amalgam, using different heavy metal formulas, have been in use. The metallic composition of amalgam from the 1950s, 1960s, and 1970s varies quite a bit from the composition used in the 1980s and 1990s because they changed the formulation, so amalgams vary. Gold has been again in vogue. Dentists often use titanium for implants, cobalt-chromium metallic partial dentures, and porcelain-fused-to-metal crowns. Those all create a little bit of a havoc as an electrical current is formed in the mouth.

YOU CAN HAVE A BATTERY IN YOUR MOUTH AND NOT EVEN KNOW IT.

In other words, you can have a battery in your mouth and not even know it.

---

40   Ibid.

41   Ibid.

My electrical engineering background gives me strong standing to understand the electrical currents that dissimilar metals can cause in the mouth. If they have dissimilar electrical charges, two metals will create a microcurrent.

It makes sense that stray electrical currents can cause the circuits not to function properly. Your most powerful electrical circuit is your brain. By placing dissimilar metals in the mouth, we are creating microcurrents that could interfere with that. Now, can that cause problems? Sure. But this galvanic reaction has another surprise: it causes the mercury in existing amalgam fillings to leach out. If you have galvanism going on, mercury can leach out, forming stains in the gum tissue called amalgam tattoos, spelling it out in neon that you have galvanism going on in your mouth. All metals in the mouth tend to tarnish over time, and we can tell when a patient has had multiple dissimilar metals in their mouth: they have more tarnish to their metal fillings. I can take one look and quickly identify a patient with galvanism, and also know that there will be an increase in the mercury being released from these amalgams, and to be watchful for signs of that genuine health risk. I have become especially attentive for Alzheimer's, multiple sclerosis, amyotrophic lateral sclerosis, and other health conditions from dental mercury exposure.

Dissimilar metals and alloys have different electrode potentials. When two or more come into contact in an electrolyte, one metal (more reactive) acts as an anode and the other (less reactive) as a cathode. With this periodic table of these various heavy metals in your mouth, you have electrical currents going on in there, inches from your brain. Combine that with mercury, and the trouble really starts. A galvanic reaction can cause mercury to come out of the fillings ten times faster than usual, which can increase mercury bioaccumulation, especially in the brain.

Electrical currents alone may cause unexplainable symptoms like anxiety, brain fog, and ringing in the ear. After having had these dissimilar metals remedied, patients reported that these symptoms diminished quickly. But the mercury build-up in the organs may create problems beyond the removal of the metal.

Mercury Detoxification

Dr. Pompa is an evangelist that bases his counseling of practitioners on a firm conviction that the crisis of modern-day allopathic medicine is the sad result of physicians chasing symptoms with medication rather than addressing the root cause of disease. His approach to getting to the "upstream cause" is what separates him from others in allopathic as well as functional medicine.

Dr. Pompa learned about mercury poisoning and detoxification the hard way.

Mad as a Hatter

"In my hours of research, when my brain was connected to reality, I came across Mad Hatters Disease and realized I was, in fact, 'mad as a hatter,'" he writes. "I had almost every symptom of this historical disease.... The term became popular because people who made felt hats, starting in the mid-1800s, became insane with a classic set of symptoms, most of which I had. As it turned out, they all had mercury poisoning."

He explains on his website that back then, mercury was used to keep down the mold population that would infiltrate and ruin the felt hats; consequently, the "mad hatters," as we alluded to earlier, "were being exposed to mercury every day, leading to their symptoms and, ultimately, their death."[42]

Pompa had a mouth full of silver fillings from the time he was young. Due to some needed dental work, he had two of them drilled out (about six remained), and gold fillings were put in their place. Even at that time, he knew silver fillings were considered harmful to the body, and gold was considered a better choice, but there was a lot more coming.

"After the fillings were replaced, I became extremely sick. Unfortunately, it took me three to four years of misery to figure out it was related to the fillings. Silver (amalgam) fillings contain 50 percent mercury, which vaporizes and cross into your brain, where it bio-accumulates."

"Changed My Life Forever"

Removing my two mercury amalgam fillings was a tragic decision that changed my life forever. However, replacing them with gold fillings while having mercury amalgam in my mouth is what I believe to be catastrophic.… they placed gold fillings and it set up a galvanic reaction (electrical current). The electrical current generated under these circumstances caused the mercury in remaining amalgam fillings to leach out at an alarming rate that would far exceed any Environmental Protection Agency (EPA) water or air quality limits several times over. I had four remaining fillings in my mouth. This unknowingly unwise decision set up the perfect storm in my mouth for heavy metal poisoning.

42   Daniel Pompa, "The Truth about Heavy Metals, Mercury Poisoning, and Mercury," POMPA, accessed September 7, 2022, https://drpompa.com/cellular-detox/detox-is-dangerous-heavy-metal-detox-mercury-toxicity-mecury-amalgam-fillings-and-mercury-poisoning.

In late 2022, the International Academy of Biological Dentistry and Medicine (IABDM) sounded the alarm on the latest published research on mercury dental amalgam using the National Health and Nutrition Examination Survey (NHANES) database, which is the "gold standard" in the world and is the only existing national survey that captures both environmental and clinical data.

The purpose of the IABDM is to promote biological dental medicine utilizing nontoxic diagnostic and therapeutic approaches in the field of clinical dentistry.

"Since the actual number of mercury dental amalgam fillings is now known, researchers David and Mark Geier have published their findings on the link between mercury dental amalgam and arthritis, asthma, and most recently mercury vapor which is a significant health risk."[43]

The researchers noted that a substantial portion of the US population is exposed to mercury vapor that exceeds the Environmental Protection Agency (EPA) limits.

In the IABDM press release, Anita Vazquez-Tibau, an international activist working to achieve a global ban on mercury stated, "Even though the US was the very first country to ratify the Minamata Convention on Mercury Treaty, the US has still not banned the use of mercury dental amalgams.… the treaty's mantra 'Make Mercury History' will never be achieved if mercury dental amalgams are not banned worldwide!"

Over 130 nations have signed the Miramata Convention. On March 26, 2022, at the fourth Conference of the Parties to the Minamata Convention on Mercury, the parties unanimously agreed to

---

43 IABDM, "Alarming Findings on Mercury Dental Amalgam," iabdm.org (International Academy of Biological Dentistry and Medicine, September 19, 2022), https://iabdm.org/alarming-findings-on-mercury-dental-amalgam/?fbclid=IwAR0sQOOym_v4ZVmLVYsl7iKeBsHr9eF-JSLIlmka-9JUHksF2M9n3GjuMYV4.

an amendment requiring countries to protect vulnerable populations from further use of dental amalgam:

"Exclude or not allow, by taking measures as appropriate, or recommend against the use of dental amalgam for the dental treatment of deciduous teeth [baby teeth], of patients under fifteen years and of pregnant and breastfeeding women."[44]

Since 2020, The US Food and Drug Administration, and Health Canada, since the 1990s, already have recommended the end of amalgam use for children and for pregnant women.

In the words of Titanic's First Officer William McMaster Murdoch, and Second Officer Charles Lightoller "women and children first."[45]

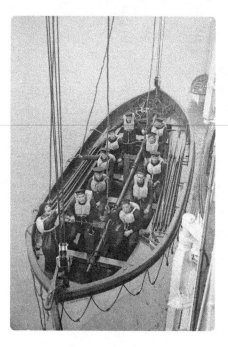

This order, also known as the Birkenhead drill, refers to a code of conduct whereby the lives of women and children were to be saved first in a life-threatening situation, typically abandoning ship, when survival resources such as lifeboats were limited.

So our cultures begin to save childbearing women and children first from the oral threat of mercury. A great start. But the rest of us are waiting for the lifeboats to be lowered.

44   WDVR, "Consumers for Dental Choice Salutes Worldwide Decision to Protect Children and Pregnant Women from Mercury Dental Fillings," https://kdvr.com/business/press-releases/cision/20220401AQ11083/consumers-for-dental-choice-salutes-worldwide-decision-to-protect-children-and-pregnant-women-from-mercury-dental-fillings/, April 1, 2022.

45   Wikipedia, "Women and Children First," https://en.wikipedia.org/wiki/Women_and_children_first, accessed September 15, 2022.

In the next chapter, I will review the unseen dangers that also exist for extractions and root canals. Exciting new holistic procedures have been developed for cleaner, safer options. We indeed have entered a whole new world of biologic dentistry, empirical and scientific, and worthy of your attention.

CLEANER, SAFER EXTRACTIONS, IMPLANTS, AND ROOT CANALS

The chances for problems go up the longer the root canal stays in your mouth because it has become a dead tooth with no blood supply to it.

If you really think about this, whole-body dentistry represents a profound, electrifying development. We have finally arrived at a place where science has recognized that each tooth has a direct connection to an organ in the body. This startling field of discovery is still quite in its infancy, and we have much to learn now that we know where to look.

Biologic dentists do things differently today. Holistic practitioners have stepped outside the status quo not to complain about general dentistry but to improve

BIOLOGIC DENTISTS DO THINGS DIFFERENTLY TODAY.

it. In this chapter, I will cover how we advance our clinical process for dealing with issues most of us will encounter as we age: root canal procedures and extractions.

We have found cleaner, safer ways to do many dental procedures and learned that by embracing the ancient Chinese wisdom of whole-body medicine, we can impact overall health in many ways. We do not look at dentistry as just the care of our teeth. We know about our meridians, these connections to critical organs in the body, and how what we do impacts that.

The Twenty-First-Century Root Canal

EARLY BEGINNINGS OF WARNINGS ABOUT ROOT CANALS

In 1925, dentist Weston A. Price (1870–1948) published a landmark article that perhaps served as the spark that ignited the bold new field of biologic dentistry.

A former director of research for the American Dental Association, Price claimed in an article for the *Journal of the American Medical Association* that "such degenerative diseases as heart troubles, kidney and bladder disorders, arthritis, rheumatism, mental illness, lung problems, and several kinds of bacterial infections arise from root canal therapy, or endodontics."

To come to this conclusion, Price conducted research (which many scientists criticize) that involved implanting teeth from the root canals of individuals with symptoms of severe heart problems and kidney disease under the skin of healthy rabbits. These same conditions arose in the rabbits, and within three days, they died. Price then implanted the same tooth in another rabbit and found a similar response, but he also found that implanting a normal extracted tooth did not affect the rabbits.[46]

Patients come in with a toothache. Usually, this indicates a severe decay problem. Perhaps an infection. Our first option is to try to save the tooth. Give it a try. In addition to the standard periapical

---

46   "Holistic Dentistry," Encyclopedia.com (Encyclopedia.com), accessed February 7, 2023, https://www.encyclopedia.com/medicine/encyclopedias-almanacs-transcripts-and-maps/holistic-dentistry.

radiograph and bite wings, we use the 3D x-ray CT scan technology to look closely at the entire root structure, be sure of our assumptions, and then we use ozone and lasers to cleanse the site, seeing if there is any hope of revival.

I believe in watchful waiting. But if the tooth becomes necrotic, there's no bringing it back to life. It's not like Frankenstein and zapping the body with electricity. We have more biocompatible materials that we can place in a tooth that traditionally we would've deemed needed a root canal to see if we can salvage the need for a deep-decayed tooth. But once it becomes really symptomatic, we usually can't save it.

Then the patient has to decide. We give them a choice. Remove it or keep basically a dead body part, a dead organ, in their body. We can extract the tooth. Or we can do a root canal procedure.

Most adults have accepted root canals in their mouth as a standard adult passage. I believe most folks think they will always be there, safely protecting the dead tooth with a cap and causing us little discomfort. The chances for problems go up the longer the root canal stays in your mouth because it has become a dead tooth with no blood supply. And it has the real potential for problems, depending on the patient's immune system and abilities to ward off any challenges from that root canal area.

Patients experiencing severe tooth pain will likely face this choice. Some will opt for a root canal, often because of aesthetics. One recent patient came in with a fractured tooth, losing about a third of the tooth toward the front. If the affected tooth affects their smile, the root canal may be the best option for quick repair. They may try them and see how it goes, and if it becomes bothersome, they will go with extraction and replacement.

Or it could be that cost plays a big part. Extraction and replacement will be more expensive and take longer.

People think root canals will last their lifetime. That would be rare. Research on this topic gets very complicated, and it has been challenging to draw a conclusive percentage success rate because of all the health and age factors and different dental situations.

But a study published in the *Journal of Applied Oral Science* in 2021, after studying 438,487 procedures in a thirteen-year retrospective study, reported success rates of endodontic therapy (root canals). The multistate outcome analysis of treatment interventions concluded that the overall survival rate was 82.8 percent.

The report also noted that "Persistent bacterial infection represents the main cause of endodontic failure. Inadequate aseptic control, missed canals, inadequate chemo-mechanical disinfection, leaking restorations, and extruded debris infected with microorganisms have all been described as causes for the persistence of bacterial infection. The human body and the infection interact constantly."[47]

So that means that 17 percent of the people can have underlying infections without any symptomatology. And then boom, they could develop systemic concerns. We regularly monitor these just as providers monitor other diseases, through radiographs deploying a 3D x-ray CT scan to make sure that changes have not occurred. Interestingly, the patient may not feel any symptoms because the nerves have died in the tooth. You may have some vague concerns or even none at all. The bacteria have a way of tricking the body. The tooth could be going in the wrong direction and can become re-abscessed. Dead teeth typically become one of the worst, if not *the* worst, sources of chronic bacterial toxicity in your body. Even antibiotics will not help in many cases because the bacteria hide protected inside your dead tooth.

47   Bhagavatula P., Moore A., Rein L., Szabo A., Ibrahim M., "Multi-State Outcome Analysis of Treatment Interventions after the Failure of Non-Surgical Root Canal Treatment: A 13-Year Retrospective Study," *Journal of Applied Oral Science*, https://www.ncbi.nlm.nih.gov/pmc/articles/PMC8425896.

CROWNS

"Because the tooth typically has a large filling or is weakened from decay, it needs to be protected from future damage and returned to normal function. We usually do this by placing a crown—a realistic-looking artificial tooth—over the tooth.

Typically made of gold, porcelain, zirconia or porcelain-fused-to-metal, crowns containing porcelain can be tinted to match the color of the other teeth. Sometimes, we insert a metal post in the tooth for structural support and to keep the crown in place if needed.

Extractions

SAVE THE TOOTH IF AT ALL POSSIBLE

Most people get their teeth taken out because of pain; they're broken. We do extractions in a more biologically predictable way. At times, we get resistance from patients about taking a tooth out because it does not hurt them. Often, these abscessed teeth do not hurt, and we have to show them the medical reasons.

The Cleveland Clinic's guidance on tooth extraction notes that dentists prefer to save natural teeth whenever possible. If the tooth has been badly damaged past the point of repair, then removal may be necessary.

The reasons for extractions include:

- Severe tooth decay (cavities)

- A fractured tooth

- An impacted tooth

- Crowded teeth

- Severe gum disease

- Tooth luxation or other dental injuries occurring when trauma, such as a fall, disrupts the tissues, ligaments, and bone that hold a tooth in place[48]

My engineering background comes into play every day because in the first few minutes of the examination, I have an idea of what the end goal should be, and I work backward from there. Then I can place in my mind all the steps to get to where I need to go, depending on their constraints.

While always thinking biologically and like a trained dentist, I study the situation from a structural point of view and a force vector point of view. That's an engineering term that refers to the push or a pull on an object and what happens when they interact. This has a vector quantity, which means it has both magnitude and direction. It may change the object's state of motion, direction, size, and shape. I look at things with one question: Will this last? Are they going to get long-term service out of it, or would I just do this to appease them? I look at patients with their best interests in mind and tell them what's really going to work and what's not right.

These forces cause me to ask, *How will things be going long term? Can I think of better options?* Recently, I had to tell a patient that we tried, but too many forces on these teeth had caused breakage and they had failed. Now we had to go to either an implant, a bridge, a partial denture, or full denture. We had to make a choice on that.

A study published in the *International Journal of Environmental Research and Public Health* reported in 2020 that 52.2 percent of tooth extractions were caused by dental cavities, with periodontal

---

48 "Tooth Extraction: Procedure, Aftercare & Recovery," www.clevelandclinic.org (Cleveland Clinic, 2021), https://my.clevelandclinic.org/health/treatments/22120-tooth-extraction.

disease representing 35.7 percent. This was a study of a relatively old adult population.[49]

Your mouth and the jaw, the angle of your teeth, and the chewing forces on them make up a significant part of my observations. I learned in engineering school that in all situations, the force vectors play a key role because we cannot have early failures when we design something. When I perform a root canal or an extraction, I know that the tooth has a direct connection to a meridian, I keep thinking aloud that this particular tooth connects to a particular organ, and I always ask questions about the patient's overall health before I get going.

If my patients have had a tough extraction, dry socket, or root canal, I become especially observant if there could be anything problematic on their meridian. Our bodies do not always reveal everything to us in black and white. We're adaptive. But I can sense the possibility that an organ could be affected here, and I make sure to inform them of that. Then we will have discussions in a follow-up visit. *Hey, did the extraction make any difference in your health?* I frequently hear the reply, *Yes, a lot.*

For anesthesia, most dentists use an array of options beginning with local anesthesia injections. The Cleveland Clinic list also includes:

- **Nitrous oxide.** Known as "laughing gas," a gas that you inhale through a mask or nosepiece. It's a good option for people who need light-level sedation. People who choose nitrous oxide usually can drive themselves to and from their appointments.

- **Oral conscious sedation.** We provide this type of sedation by mouth, usually in pill form, about an hour before your dental appointment. Common medications used for this purpose

---

49   P.C. Passarelli, S. Pagnoni, G.B. Piccirillo, V. Desantis, M. Benegiamo, A Liguori, R. Papa, P. Papi, G. Pompa, A. D'Addona, "Reasons for Tooth Extractions and Related Risk Factors in Adult Patients: A Cohort Study," *International Journal of Environmental Research and Public Health,* https://www.ncbi.nlm.nih.gov/pmc/articles/PMC7178127/.

include diazepam, midazolam, triazolam, and lorazepam. Oral conscious sedation can be used on its own or in combination with nitrous oxide or intravenous sedation. People who choose oral conscious sedation will need a friend or family member to drive them to and from their appointment.

- **Intravenous (IV) sedation.** We use this for people with significant dental anxiety or for those undergoing lengthy procedures. We deliver sedative and pain medications—such as midazolam and meperidine—directly to your bloodstream using an IV line.[50]

PREPARING FOR AN IMPLANT AND BONE GRAFTING

Most typical extractions are done with the goal of just removing the tooth and this may not go far enough. A biologic extraction, as I refer to it, often requested by educated patients, takes a lot of skill and patience to minimize hard and soft tissue injury. The area will often be bone grafted, which basically is a scaffold for the body, so the area does not collapse in width and in height. If the area starts collapsing, then we lose the volume of bone for an ideal implant placement.

The kinds of grafts available include animal bone, human cadaver bone, and the patient's own bone, but we must harvest that with another surgery. Or we can use synthetics, or collagen parts, and then we can use the patient's own blood to form a matrix, to start the healing process, and minimize dry sockets or problems from the extraction. We use the body's own cells to promote a healthier environment for things to start reproducing and produce bone. This faster way occurs by using your own blood as a graft material.

---

50   Ibid.

When my son was born, we arranged for a sample of his cord blood to be saved. I had it frozen. Eric has stem cells from blood in case it is needed. But we cannot use stored blood for this type of procedure. We take the blood, just like a normal phlebotomist would take blood from the back of your hand or at the crux of your elbow. We borrow a few vials of blood for the procedure, spinning it down in a centrifuge, which creates a condensed collection of cells. After a few minutes at a certain RPM and time, the blood cells separate, ready to put into the extracted site.

As it separates in the centrifuge, we can use the cells as graft material and put it in the socket site to help pump up the tissues or to accelerate tissue growth. We can also use an injectable portion of that to make what we call "sticky bone." It becomes just another type of membrane used to help with the healing and covering of the wound site. This PRF (platelet-rich fibrin), 100 percent natural, helps protect the bony surgical site from infection, accelerates the healing process, and decreases pain after the procedure.

Just after the extraction, we scrape the walls in the extraction site to get back to the bone. We scrape out this periodontal ligament. Sometimes a surgical round bur is needed. I use ozone water to help irrigate and remove some of the infectious areas. We're trying to remove the granulation tissue and any infected areas, deep, deep down inside. I find with this ozone water that the infected area or the granulation tissue removes much more easily. Ozone water also has an angiogenesis property that stimulates blood vessel formation. Then we just scrape it all out and make sure to get back to some good solid bone and make sure it has some blood from the walls of the extraction site.

After clearing the space out, I use my Fotona laser, setting a program on it for socket sterilization. Unlike the Star Wars-type laser, this wonderful tool concentrates light energy from a wand with a small fiber optic. I place it into the socket, through a fiber optic tube, and it cleans up the area, and it helps sterilize it further. The energy from the laser works reliably because of the porous bone property, which helps spread the energy laterally, as we want to reduce infection and inflammation. We want to promote good blood formation and to cover the area to protect it from bacteria. When we do all that, we have an ideal environment in which the body can grow its own bone. Then we can use that area for future implants, if necessary.

We make a PRF membrane and suture it over the top of everything to hold our graft in there and to protect the wound site. It becomes fabulously self-contained and protected. This transforms into solid bone, without using anything artificial or something the patient may not want.

"Almost Magical"

A lengthy procedure, this kind of biologic dentistry extraction can take more time and skill than a typical extraction. It takes five minutes to draw the blood. It takes fifteen minutes for the blood clot to form. The patient cannot come in ahead. We do not store blood, requiring everything to be done at the appointment. At times, I will have a phlebotomist come into the office to help out with the really difficult blood draws. Typically, I describe the healing through the PRF as almost magical. We really rarely have any complications.

THE HEALING THROUGH PRF IS ALMOST MAGICAL. WE RARELY HAVE ANY COMPLICATIONS.

Some patients have the idea that they want an extraction, and they want to think about an implant later. Some people want an extraction, and they want an implant put in right away. We call this an immediate-placed implant. Both offer wonderful procedures to do with predictability. Many practitioners recommend extracting the tooth, grafting, and then having the patient come back in four months and do another CT scan. Then do the implant surgery. But if a patient wants a procedure done on the same day, then we can do both extraction and an implant. The immediate implant process can save the patient four months and surgery.

A Dental Implant Surgery

Dental exam: Before the implant process begins, we conduct a thorough exam using the 3D x-ray CT scan. Not having to rely solely on two-dimensional x-rays helps to better assess your dental health, especially the bone that will support the implant.

Removal of tooth or teeth: We then remove the tooth or teeth affected.

Bone graft: If the initial exam shows insufficient bone to support the implant, we will need to perform a bone graft, where needed. A waiting period is needed for the bone to mature.

Insertion of implant: We place the implant itself into place in the jawbone. This also requires a period of healing afterward. (We may perform these two surgeries, extraction and implant placement, at the same time.) The implant becomes an artificial tooth root. We anchor it deep into the bone, just like a natural tooth. As the healing from the implantation begins and bone grows around the new implant, the patient will wear a temporary, removable denture to cover the gap where the original tooth was taken out.

Abutment added: After two or three months, when enough bone has grown in to stabilize, we add the part of the implant that will hold the crown in place—the abutment—and close the gum area around its edges. Now, the gum needs to heal, which can take four to six weeks.

Crown inserted: In the final step, we place the crown, custom manufactured to match the color, shape, and size of the other teeth. We do this by making molds or digital impressions of existing teeth and jaw after placing the abutment.[51]

We can delay the implant procedure for nine or ten months, but after that time, the body starts reducing the bone volume, making an ideal implant placement less predictable.

WebMD reports that success rates of dental implants vary, depending on where in the jaw the implants are placed, but in general, "dental implants have a success rate of up to 98 percent. With proper care, implants can last a lifetime."[52]

In our next chapter on children's and adolescent dentistry, I offer my views on the overuse of fluoride and the general epidemic of pulling every wisdom tooth in every mouth on the planet, and some advanced thinking on other aspects of our children's dental journey.

51   Anne Russell, "Dental Implants: Everything You Need to Know," forbes.com (*Forbes*, February 1, 2023), https://www.forbes.com/health/body/dental-implants-guide/.

52   "Dental Implants: Surgery, Advantages, Risks, and Insurance Questions," WebMD.com (WebMD, July 30, 2021), https://www.webmd.com/oral-health/guide/dental-implants#091e9c5e80007bac-1-4.

OUR KIDS: UNNECESSARY WISDOM TOOTH REMOVAL, THE OVERUSE OF FLUORIDE, AND MORE

Each year, despite the risks of any surgical procedure, millions of healthy, asymptomatic wisdom teeth are extracted from young patients in the United States ...

I suppose it may be overstating it to call the disquieting plague of wisdom tooth removal an *epidemic*.

Wisdom tooth extraction refers to the surgical procedure to remove one or more wisdom teeth—the four permanent adult teeth located at the back corners of your mouth on the top and bottom. But this tendency to see a wisdom tooth and immediately take action to remove it, in my view, seems about 90 percent unnecessary or premature. Are wisdom teeth problematic? I am a minimalist when it comes to surgical interven-

ARE WISDOM TEETH PROBLEMATIC? MOST OF MY PATIENTS GET ALONG FINE WITH WISDOM TEETH, EVEN IF IMPACTED.

tions. Most of my patients get along fine with wisdom teeth, even if impacted (teeth that do not break through but stay in the gums.)

In many people, wisdom teeth do not break through the gum and grow out—or only part of them do. Most young adults have at least one wisdom tooth that has not broken through, a situation more common in the lower jaw than in the upper jaw, usually because of a lack of space. Other teeth may then get in the way of the wisdom tooth. It might come in crooked.

MAYO CLINIC, WISDOM TOOTH EXTRACTION

Practitioners may recommend removal of that impacted wisdom tooth if it could result in problems such as

- Pain.
- Trapping food and debris behind the wisdom tooth.
- Infection or gum disease (periodontal disease).
- Tooth decay in a partially erupted wisdom tooth.
- Damage to a nearby tooth or surrounding bone.
- Development of a fluid-filled sac (cyst) around the wisdom tooth.
- Complications with orthodontic treatments to straighten other teeth.
- Preventing future dental problems.[53]

The *New York Times* published an article years ago titled "Wisdom of Having That Tooth Removed," which summed it up well.

"Each year, despite the risks of any surgical procedure, millions of healthy, asymptomatic wisdom teeth are extracted from young patients in the United States, often as they prepare to leave for college. Many dental plans cover the removal of these teeth, which have partly grown in or are impacted below the gum," said reporter Roni Caryn Rabin.

---

53   "Wisdom Tooth Extraction," mayoclinic.org (Mayo Foundation for Medical Education and Research, January 31, 2018), https://www.mayoclinic.org/tests-procedures/wisdom-tooth-extraction/about/pac-20395268.

"But," she continues, "scientific evidence supporting the routine prophylactic extraction of wisdom teeth is surprisingly scant, and in some countries, the practice has been abandoned. 'Everybody is at risk for appendicitis, but do you take out everyone's appendix?' said Dr. Greg J. Huang, chairperson of orthodontics at the University of Washington in Seattle. 'I'm not against removing wisdom teeth, but you should do an assessment and have a good clinical reason.'"[54]

There are no scientifically proven health benefits of pulling wisdom teeth that do not cause any problems. Wisdom teeth, or third molars, are the last permanent teeth to appear (erupt) in the mouth. These teeth usually appear between the ages of seventeen and twenty-five. Some people never develop wisdom teeth. For others, wisdom teeth erupt normally—just as their other molars did—and cause no problems.

The Teeth That Nobody Seems to Want

I've changed my opinion on wisdom tooth removal over the years. Years ago, I thought everybody who did not have enough space in their mouth should have their wisdom teeth extracted.

More recently, I have changed my tune. Instead of removal, I promote the early development of proper breathing, tongue posture, and expansion orthodontics (instead of just orthodontics for aesthetics), which I refer to as *nonextraction orthodontics*.

> *"But if you can keep a wisdom tooth in there, you're better off in the long run, in my opinion."*

---

54   Roni Caryn Rabin, "Wisdom of Having That Tooth Removed," nytimes.com (*New York Times*, September 5, 2011), https://www.nytimes.com/2011/09/06/health/06consumer.html#:~:text=Another%20 expert%2C%20Dr.,acknowledged%20that%20data%20is%20limited.

For decades, many of us had practiced with the belief that our culture has evolved to have smaller jaws, unable to fully accommodate all thirty-two teeth. A September 2020 journal article in *Bioscience* explains why we have more crooked teeth than ever. Surprisingly, jaw shrinkage since the agricultural revolution has led to an epidemic of crooked teeth, a lack of adequate space for the last molars (wisdom teeth), and constricted airways, a major cause of sleep-related stress.

Despite claims that genetics represent the cause of this jaw epidemic, "the speed with which human jaws have changed, especially in the last few centuries, happened much too quickly to be evolutionary. "Virtually all aspects of how modern people function, and rest, are radically different from those of our ancestors," the journal noted.[55]

Once we accept that narrow jaws and malocclusion are environmental rather than genetic, the focus of orthodontic treatment necessarily changes from the easy route of extracting teeth to the optimal solution of expanding the jaw to accommodate the teeth.

A movement grows across the developed world against this wholesale removal of wisdom teeth. Ashley Craig, one such vocal opponent who campaigns against unnecessary wisdom tooth extractions, makes a great point when he reminds us that we do not have our appendix removed unless it causes us problems.

"Why, then, do nearly 85 percent of adults go through the trauma of surgery for teeth that frequently remain dormant in the bone, or even erupt fully with no issue? Critics of routine extraction cite many studies, among them one that found complications occurred for only 12 percent of 1,756 middle-aged people who did not have their wisdom teeth removed."[56]

55   S. Kahn, P. Ehrlich, M. Feldman, R. Sapolsky, S. Won, "The Jaw Epidemic: Recognition, Origins, Cures, and Prevention," *Bioscience*, (July 2020), https://www.ncbi.nlm.nih.gov/pmc/articles/PMC7498344/.

56   Ashley Craig, "Extractions & the Airway," righttogrow.org (Right to Grow), accessed February 7, 2023, https://www.righttogrow.org/extractions_the_airway.

Many of us get along fine without our wisdom teeth. The body has a better chance of having the wisdom tooth erupt properly if the jaws are wide enough for it. But if you can keep a wisdom tooth in there, you're better off in the long run, in my opinion.

Over almost thirty years of practice, I have seen very few patients that had to have them removed because they were cystic later in life. And that's the argument, that you're going to have a higher risk by waiting until adulthood.

You may be taking drugs, such as blood thinners, in your sixties and seventies. It makes it more complicated to have an extraction and heal properly or heal with fewer issues, as compared to having them out as a teenager or in your early twenties.

My older sons came along when I was among the vast number of dentists who recommended extraction. We removed their wisdom teeth. My youngest son Eric (eleven years younger than my oldest), we have managed differently by developing his arches so we can have at least a potential of not having the extractions done.

Most people don't want their wisdom teeth out. Most people don't want any surgery done, especially in their teen years or twenties. They're like, *no way.*

MAYO CLINIC

An impacted wisdom tooth may

- Grow at an angle toward the next tooth (second molar).
- Grow at an angle toward the back of the mouth.
- Grow at a right angle to the other teeth, as if the wisdom tooth is "lying down" within the jawbone.
- Grow straight up or down like other teeth but stay trapped within the jawbone.[57]

---

57   Ibid.

Wisdom teeth seldom offer easy removal. If it were easy and risk-free, I might have a different viewpoint on the issue.

The Mayo Clinic

During a wisdom tooth extraction, your dentist or oral surgeon

- Makes an incision in the gum tissue to expose the tooth and bone.

- Removes bone that blocks access to the tooth root.

- Divides the tooth into sections if it's easier to remove in pieces.

- Removes the tooth.

- Cleans the site of the removed tooth of any debris from the tooth or bone.

- Stitches the wound closed to promote healing, though this isn't always necessary.

- Places gauze over the extraction site to control bleeding and to help a blood clot form.[58]

It's not just me. Thousands of dental specialists disagree about the value of extracting impacted wisdom teeth that aren't causing problems (asymptomatic).

It's difficult to predict future problems with impacted wisdom teeth. However, here's what the Mayo Clinic lists as the rationale for preventive extraction:

- Symptom-free wisdom teeth could still harbor disease.

- If there isn't enough space for the tooth to erupt, it's often hard to get to it and clean it properly.

---

58   Ibid.

- Serious complications with wisdom teeth happen less often in younger adults.

- Older adults may experience difficulty with surgery and complications after surgery.

Most wisdom tooth extractions do not result in long-term complications. However, removal of impacted wisdom teeth occasionally requires a surgical approach that involves making an incision in the gum tissue and removing bone. Rarely, complications can include:

- Painful dry socket, or exposure of bone when the post-surgical blood clot is lost from the site of the surgical wound (socket).

- Infection in the socket from bacteria or trapped food particles.

- Damage to nearby teeth, nerves, jawbone, or sinuses.[59]

The main goal of a holistic or biologic dentist will always be to keep us safe from harmful substances and to avoid inflicting harm at all costs. *First, do no harm.*

Our Everyday Fluoride

What diseases are the most common in the world? Infections probably come to mind. Or heart disease, or cancer, or perhaps even AIDS. Actually, it is the common cold! And what comes in second? Tooth decay![60]

Cavities are unsightly and can cause pain. But poor oral health can also allow bacteria to enter the bloodstream and precipitate respiratory or heart problems. Luckily, though, we can prevent tooth decay.

---

59   Ibid.

60   Joe Schwarcz, "The Fluoride Controversy," mcgill.ca (Office for Science and Society, March 20, 2017), https://www.mcgill.ca/oss/article/health/fluoride-controversy.

Proper oral hygiene and reducing sweets in the diet work as does making the teeth more resistant to decay by chemical intervention.

We now arrive at the topic of fluoride. A good friend and I had a polite argument about this recently. Now, no ordinary patient, she serves as a science writer.

We were sitting at a picnic table at Boy Scout summer camp, and we started talking about fluoride; she mentioned the fact that she is quite supportive of the use of fluoride. And I'm like, *Oh, do you know what? I really don't write prescriptions for fluoride because it may lower the IQ of the child, potentially.*

SOME RESEARCHERS NOW QUESTION WHETHER LOW DOSES OF FLUORIDE CAN HAVE EFFECTS, INCLUDING A DIP IN IQ IN CHILDREN EXPOSED TO IT IN UTERO.

Some toxicologists and epidemiologists now question whether even low doses of fluoride can have systemic effects, including causing a dip in IQ in children who were exposed to it *in utero.* It's an emotional topic.

That got her attention. And she says, *No, that's not true; it reduces decay rates.*

I said, *It really doesn't reduce decay rates. Look at the graphs; countries that are fluoridated and not fluoridated … not much difference.*

Talk about a standoff. I do fully agree with many major aspects of her argument about fluoride.

So does the American Academy of Pediatrics. An updated clinical report covers caries prevention in primary care, which was issued on November 30, 2020: "Dental caries remains the most common chronic disease of childhood in the United States. Cavities are a largely preventable condition, and fluoride has proven effectiveness in caries prevention."[61]

The article describes that the development of cavities requires four components: teeth, bacteria, carbohydrate exposure, and time.

"Once teeth emerge, they become colonized with cariogenic bacteria. The bacteria metabolize carbohydrates and create acid as a byproduct. The acid dissolves the mineral content of enamel (demineralization) and, over time, with repeated acid attacks, the enamel surface disintegrates and results in a cavity in the tooth."

Protective factors that help to remineralize enamel include exposing the teeth to fluoride and limiting the frequency of carbohydrate consumption (to three meals and two healthy snacks per day).

The Academy news release mentions choosing less cariogenic foods (selecting cheese or raw carrots over candy or crackers; selecting fresh fruit over dried fruit or processed fruit snacks), practicing good oral hygiene (brushing twice a day for two minutes and flossing between all teeth that touch), and receiving regular dental assessments and care."[62]

Solid science. But we have no choice in the matter unless we use water that has been specifically filtered for fluoride exclusively. Here's a question for you. What parts per million (ppm) or milligrams per liter of fluoride does your community add to your water? Most folks look like "a deer in headlights" when I ask that question.

The Centers for Disease Control and Prevention (CDC) reports that in 2018, 73 percent of the US population that benefited from

61   "American Academy of Pediatrics: Fluoride Remains a Powerful Tool to Prevent Tooth Decay," aap. org (American Academy of Pediatrics, November 30, 2020), https://www.aap.org/en/news-room/news-releases/aap/2020/american-academy-of-pediatrics-fluoride-remains-a-powerful-tool-to-prevent-tooth-decay/.

62   Melinda Clark et. al, "Fluoride Use in Caries Prevention in the Primary Care Setting," Publications.aap. org (American Academy of Pediatrics, December 1, 2020), https://publications.aap.org/pediatrics/article/146/6/e2020034637/33536/Fluoride-Use-in-Caries-Prevention-in-the-Primary.

community water systems, or 207,426,535 people, had access to fluoridated water.[63]

Especially with young adults, their nutritional status has a great bearing on decay prevention.

The tubules of the tooth (from inside the tooth) flow out like a fountain to prevent the bacteria with a pH-neutral to alkaline environment, as compared to an acidic environment, which sucks in fluids, which contain bacteria, and then it causes decay. It's almost as simple as that. If we correct the nutritional status, then we won't need fluoride, and that's my stance on it.

Tooth enamel is mostly composed of hydroxyapatite, a substance readily damaged by acids. Naturally occurring bacteria in the mouth, streptococcus mutans in particular, feed on sugars, metabolize these to acids, and presto, cavities appear. However, if fluoride supplements the diet, or topically applied to the teeth, it gets incorporated into the structure of the tooth, forming a more acid-stable substance called fluoroapatite.[64]

I haven't written a prescription for systemic fluoride for a child in a decade. Maybe there are some clinical applications of the use of fluoride, I buy that to halt the progression of decay in senior citizens, and it might show some efficacy short term for children if it's applied topically in the chair, but not systemically and not every night using fluoridated toothpaste.

Just recently, I changed my family to nonfluoridated toothpaste. I do not believe that our body has such a lack of fluoride that we need systemic supplementation. I followed the American Dental Association's recommendations for my first two children up to a certain age,

---

63   "Water Fluoridation Data & Statistics," cdc.gov (Centers for Disease Control and Prevention, August 28, 2020), https://www.cdc.gov/fluoridation/statistics/index.htm.

64   Joe Schwarcz, "The Fluoride Controversy," mcgill.ca (Office for Science and Society, March 20, 2017), https://www.mcgill.ca/oss/article/health/fluoride-controversy.

where I made sure they had their fluoride tablets and their fluoride rinses. I followed suit.

Then when I became a little bit smarter, I realized that I was doing my children and the children in my practice a disservice by writing prescriptions for fluoride tablets. I started discussing things with the parents more about their diet and, of course, their brushing habits versus trying to provide a magic pill that's going to prevent them from getting decay.

Because typically they do get decay even though taking fluoride tablets. If you don't take them the right way or take too many, problems can develop with the teeth, even adult teeth, where they can have too much fluoride incorporated in them.

Then you develop these unsightly mottling of their teeth, these brown or white spots on their teeth. It's just a structural change of the tooth enamel, and it actually, in the long term, makes the tooth weaker.

The studies I've read suggest that systemic fluoride may not be an ideal situation. You can potentially develop early calcification of glands, and you can actually have a decrease in the child's IQ. That sounds like an alarm, but an actively building theory somewhat validated in some global studies.

In a recent Canadian study of fluoride exposure from infant formula, it was shown that exposure to increasing levels of fluoride in tap water was associated with diminished nonverbal intellectual abilities; the effect was more pronounced among formula-fed children.[65]

---

65   Christine Till, Rivka Green, David Flora, Richard Hornung, E. Angeles Martinez-Mier, Maddy Blazer, Linda Farmus, Pierre Ayotte, Gina Muckle, Bruce Lanphear, National Library of Medicine, "Fluoride Exposure from Infant Formula and Child IQ in a Canadian Birth Cohort," https://pubmed. ncbi.nlm.nih.gov/31743803/, January 2020, accessed September 20, 2022.

The *Washington Post* writer Ben Guarino authored an article entitled "Study Raises Questions about Fluoride and Children's IQ," cautioning us not to react too quickly.

"A study of young children in Canada suggests those whose mothers drank fluoridated tap water while pregnant had slightly lower IQ scores than children whose mothers lived in nonfluoridated cities.

"But don't dash for the nearest bottled water yet. Health experts at the American Academy of Pediatrics and the American Dental Association cautioned that public policy and drinking water consumption should not change on the basis of this study."[66]

I do not particularly like fluoride in the water system, because first of all, we don't have a choice.

You'd have to use a reverse osmosis filter system to remove it. We don't even know how much fluoride we're getting from bottled waters or when visiting another community, much less the content added to our tap water. You may get topical fluoride painted on your teeth. The studies show this could be of some benefit, but not for very long. It's not lasting, and there's a lot of swallowing of it. I remember when I was doing fluoride in the dental office, I would put gel fluoride in these trays and the patient would stick them in their mouth for three or four minutes. Some children would reflexively swallow the fluoride, causing them to vomit. If you read the back of a toothpaste tube, it says, *do not swallow, highly toxic*. If a child swallows a whole tube of toothpaste, assuming it's paste candy, then they could potentially die from it. That's how highly toxic it is.

So for me, it's used sparingly in the right situations, not necessarily for children, even though parents want it, but I think parents can be educated. Holistic folks and those more educated about the potential harm it can do, don't want it. Because I'm in a practice with another dentist and all hygienists are school-trained to place fluoride on patients, we have an agreement to have a discussion with the parents to make sure they understand the issues, but we just don't automatically do it.

How Much Is Too Much?

FLUORIDE-CONTAINING DENTIFRICES SUCH AS TOOTHPASTE, PROFESSIONALLY USED VARNISHES/GELS, AND MOUTH RINSES

Fluoride toothpastes are available as low fluoride (500 ppm), standard fluoride (1,100–1,500 ppm), and high-fluoride toothpaste (greater than 1,500 ppm).

Fluoride is added in different forms to toothpaste and mouth rinses such as sodium fluoride, mono-fluorophosphate, or stannous fluoride.

The mouth rinses have an advantage over toothpaste because of their low viscosity, which results in better delivery to the least accessible areas of the teeth such as pits and fissures and interproximal areas.[67]

In recent years, we all cued up for fluoridated toothpaste. We get fluoridated mouthwash. Processed foods and beverages are made with fluoridated water. Then we add fluoride to our tap water. Some segments of the population may be exposed to more than the optimal amount of fluoride. It is also quite clear that due to these sources of fluoride, as well as to earlier and better dental care, the gap in the incidence of cavities between fluoridated and nonfluoridated areas has narrowed considerably. But at what cost?

---

67   Rizwan Ullah, Muhammad Sohail Zafar, and Nazish Shahani, "Potential Fluoride Toxicity from Oral Medicaments: A Review," https://www.ncbi.nlm.nih.gov/ (U.S. National Library of Medicine, August 2017), https://www.ncbi.nlm.nih.gov/pmc/articles/PMC5651468/.

Fluoride is a poison. Toxicity is always a question of dose! But that is elusive. There is no one source to seek out to get information on fluoridation. It's just a free-for-all. I remember the commercials in the sixties about fluoridation and oral care products.

Now, it has jumped to the younger generations. Young people don't even think about any possible negative effects of too much fluoride.

I watch international studies. Pretty much everywhere, the decay rate difference between fluoridated nations and nonfluoridated nations narrows more every year. And I know it has to do with diet.

I like the International Academy of Oral Medicine & Toxicology (IAOMT) website. They may be biased against a lot of things, but I really think they're scientific in their approach.

This advocacy organization summarizes the fluoride controversy clearly.

"Sources of human exposure to fluoride have drastically increased since community water fluoridation began in the US in the 1940s. In addition to water, these sources now include food, air, soil, pesticides, fertilizers, dental products used at home and in the dental office, pharmaceutical drugs, cookware (nonstick Teflon), and an array of other consumer items used on a regular basis. Most people are not aware of important fluoride facts about these sources."[68]

The (IAOMT) website also notes that researchers suspect that exposure to fluoride could impact nearly every part of the human body, and the potential for harm has been clearly established in scientific research. A 2006 report by the National Research Council (NRC) identified a number of health risks associated with fluoride exposure. "Susceptible sub-populations, such as infants, children, and individuals with diabetes or renal or thyroid problems, are known

---

68   David Kennedy and Griffin Cole, "Fluoride Facts: Sources, Exposure and Health Effects," https:// iaomt.org/ (International Academy of Oral Medicine and Technology, January 13, 2023), https:// iaomt.org/resources/fluoride-facts/.

to be more severely impacted by the intake of fluoride. Since such populations and all people can potentially be impacted by fluoride exposure, consumers need to know these crucial fluoride facts."

"Perhaps we should wait the requisite 150 years,
as with the use of mercury in the mouth,
to reluctantly admit that maybe we missed something
for fifteen decades."

I don't do fluoride on everybody. I do not place sealants on everybody. I'd rather discuss nutrition with the parents than apply something that coats their teeth and gives them a false sense that they have an impenetrable coating and that they can consume from all food groups. And I'm saying that soda and candy are not a food group.

Tongue-Tie

Orthodontics, a wonderful thing for children, should be done with an open mind and not just for the aesthetics, but with the view that we have an opportunity to improve the health of a child through proper mouth expansion.

We need to identify this early on in a patient, and I'm not talking about tongue-tie, which has to be identified even earlier, and not just because they're not latching on, but they just don't have the freedom.

Some babies are born with tongue-tie, also known as ankyloglossia, a condition which limits their tongue movements. Your tongue needs to be able to reach almost every part of your mouth. That full range of motion enables different sounds when you speak. It also helps you swallow and sweep away bits of food to keep your mouth clean.

WebMD explains the problem with babies with tongue-tie as a problem with the lingual frenulum. That's the small stretch of tissue that connects the underside of your tongue to the bottom of your mouth. It might be too short and tight or attached way up near the tip of the tongue. Either way, it ties the tongue in place. For some, it's not much of an issue. For others, it can lead to problems with breastfeeding. Later on, it can affect eating and speaking.[69]

It narrows the palette. And it narrows the mid-face. And eventually, it narrows the airway. That creates speech issues, swallowing issues, and an improper form of the palette. We all need to be acutely aware of a child's exam early on when a dialogue with the parents should begin, ideally within the first year. If they're having a problem breastfeeding, we want to see them to identify if there's a tongue-tie issue.

I know lactation nurses are quite aware of that, which is awesome, then we can begin our work early. We really want to see them by their first birthday with the parent, of course, to see how they are developing orally, and structurally, if they have bad habits with pacifiers or the tongue. But we also want to check their palettes and nutrition to ensure what they're eating contributes to facial growth. Nutrition and food densities are very important as they mature.

We have found that children that just eat the pureed-type food, the baby food in the jars, aren't masticating the food. They're just swallowing it and not actually strengthening their jaw, because by strengthening the jaw muscles, the child strengthens and develops facial growth.

Many children are identified for orthodontia needs later rather than sooner. Some people advocate even at age three, to help with the transverse, the lateral growth of a child through different modalities.

It can be difficult to manage children through this process at age three or four. So, often, we wait until kindergarten or first grade to try to put them into some sort of expansion appliance.

---

69   William Moore, "Tongue-Tie in Babies (Ankyloglossia)," WebMD.com (WebMD, August 14, 2022), https://www.webmd.com/children/tongue-tie-babies.

That's not the perfect world, perhaps a few years too late. If we pass that stage of recognition, the child develops crooked teeth because there's a lack of room in the jaw for the teeth. I think we've missed a great opportunity for facial growth. Orthodontics needs to be considered in facial growth development, helping to direct the bone structure to develop in a proper manner.

We cannot underestimate the importance of the way patients chew and swallow their food and how they swallow their own saliva, and the proper placement of the tongue up to the palate, helps develop the width of the face.

Developing the width of the face not only develops the airway at the base of your skull, but it also develops the mid-face, the nasal area. That will mature into better nasal breathing instead of mouth breathing. There's a lot to it in recognition early on, but it challenges parents to send their kids for braces super-early for a lot of reasons. Financially, the insurance companies will usually pay for one round of orthodontics. A lot of orthopedics, and facial bone structural growth needs to occur before the teeth get straightened.

It can be a dual pathway between orthopedics and the growth of the bone. If the jawbone has proper width, it results in good lip support, meaning that the child has not become a mouth breather, but rather a nasal breather. You have proper swallowing. The teeth should just fall into place. Isn't that amazing? If we establish good nutrition, eating dense foods that include meat and vegetables, many things go right.

Chewing strongly, breathing properly, and you don't have your mouth wide open at night snoring or having nasal issues, the child's face starts to grow the proper way. The teeth are going to fit. We try to improve upon the width of the arch with proper lip function, enclosure, and better nasal breathing.

Braces and Clear Aligners

No child wants traditional orthodontics when they're sixteen or seventeen years old. Today we have alternatives. We can use clear retainers and clear aligners that do very much the same thing as wire braces, and the kids love it.

Putting braces on when a child reaches ten or eleven, in my view, opens the door for problems. If they have a late growth spurt, then they have malocclusion all over again. They never correct the issue because the braces were put on too early, and they may not have developed the arches properly for future growth. I prefer later orthodontics for aesthetics, but early intervention for proper orthopedics, for facial growth.

A lot of children need to be put in traditional metal-type braces because of compliance. The clear aligners actually cost a little more, but clear aligners, in most cases, accomplish the same thing as traditional wires. We are now using aligner therapy for expansion and airway solutions. It's really an aesthetic decision for teens. And now most kids opt for the clear aligner route.

We're also using clear aligners for adults because adults don't want to be in the traditional railroad tracks, they want something they can take out if they're on a Zoom call or a conference call. There are a lot of newscasters early in their careers, and even the veterans, getting clear aligners. We cannot tell on TV that they have them in. It's very aesthetic, and it's very speech oriented. I like them. The kids stay motivated and compliance with that is very, very high. Kids will just not lose them because it costs money when you lose a tray. (You must get it remanufactured.) But I think most children, and teenagers, take the alignment seriously and are compliant.

The innovation in clear aligners impresses me. They have a program now called CandidPro, which limits the needed visits to the office. CandidPro begins like other orthodontic treatments: with a consultation with the dentist or orthodontist. They evaluate your teeth to see if you are a candidate for orthodontics. If you are, they will send a scan to the CandidPro office, where the advanced computer will assess the precise tooth movements necessary to achieve the straight smile you desire. Then the computer will break those movements up into a set of steps. It makes a clear plastic aligner to achieve each of these steps. Then CandidPro will ship you the aligner kit, including the full set of aligners and the monitoring tool.

Patients wear each aligner for at least twenty-two hours a day for about two weeks, checking in periodically with the monitoring tool. This is an attachment for a cell phone that lets the camera take a detailed image of your teeth. This is sent to your dental office and CandidPro to evaluate the progress of the treatment. If your treatment is progressing, you move on to your next aligner. You can go from start to finish through video, and not in the chair. That's a really cool thing, a wonderful choice with new technology. I have several of those cases going on now.

Could this be the end of wire braces? Do we see the cusp of the end of that? Probably not. Complexity, compliance, and finances are the three reasons why we would go the traditional way. But these new clear aligners represent a game changer in my mind, for now. More innovations are coming. But everybody wants clear aligners if given a choice by Mom.

This topic has been all about prevention. Our next topic covers some of the things that can go very wrong, very quickly. These next issues are hard to see coming, like a powerful jab.

CHAPTER 6:

THE CONNECTIONS BETWEEN YOUR JAW, TEETH, TMJ, AND SLEEP

This can be a big deal. We use our TMJ at least 2,000 times a day, the Champ probably even more ...

When it's working well, our jaw is a marvel of mobility.

It usually works great, and when it's not, it affects everything, and you will probably rush to the doctor or dentist. Sometimes there is minimal warning.

The temporomandibular joints (TMJ) are the two joints that connect your lower jaw to your skull. More specifically, they are the joints that slide and rotate in front of each ear. They consist of the mandible (the lower jaw) and the temporal bone (the side and base of the skull).

It can be a big deal. We use our TMJ at least two thousand times a day.[70] There may be pain. There may be an incomplete jaw opening.

---

70   Mieszko Wieckiewicz, Klaus Boening, Piotr Wiland, Yuh-Yuan Shiau, Anna Paradowska-Stolarz, "Reported Concepts for the Treatment Modalities and Pain Management of Temporomandibular Disorders," *The Journal of Headache and Pain*, (December 7, 2014), https://thejournalofheadache-andpain.biomedcentral.com/articles/10.1186/s10194-015-0586-5.

Your jaw can make noises, they can pop, and you can become engulfed in radiating facial pain or get headaches from it. Not a lot of fun. A battery of emotions arises. *What is happening to me?*

The Champ

As a nine-year-old Tenderfoot Boy Scout, when our group gathered, we would talk about sports, and one of the most memorable sporting events was the March 31, 1973, title bout between Muhammad Ali and Ken Norton. The reason I mention this comes from the news that the Champ suffered a badly broken jaw from Ken Norton's fist during the fight. Ali had entered the ring as Champion of the World, wearing a sequin-encrusted white robe given to him by Elvis Presley. With very little ring experience, Norton was supposed to be a punching dummy.

I remember my scouting friends' reaction when we learned that Ali had a broken jaw. Nobody knew until after the fight when they rushed him to the hospital for a ninety-minute operation, leaving him with his mouth wired shut for weeks. Ali reported little pain during the bout, but his corner noticed the increased blood flow from his mouthpiece. Announcer Howard Cosell called for Ali to retire.

People who suffer from a broken jaw may develop numbness in their lower lip, chin, or tongue. A series of nerves run through the mandible, and certain fractures can impede these nerves. Unfortunately, if the nerves are affected and you do not get proper treatment, it can affect your speech in the long term. People who have broken a jaw are prone to TMJ disorders.

Interestingly, the Champ could still talk trash after the fight, seemingly without his lips moving, through clenched teeth, like a ventriloquist.

The TMJ is one of the most complex joints in the body. A solid jawbone connects two freely hinged joints, and it's supposed to move vertically up and down and laterally side to side.

Johns Hopkins Medicine notes that when the mandible and the joints are correctly aligned, smooth muscle actions, such as chewing, talking, yawning, and swallowing, can take place.[71] When these structures (muscles, ligaments, disk, jawbone, temporal bone) do not align, or they do not synchronize in movement, problems occur.

The National Institute of Dental and Craniofacial Research classifies TMD by the following:

Myofascial pain. The most common form of TMD refers to discomfort or pain in the fascia (connective tissue covering the muscles) and muscles controlling jaw, neck, and shoulder function.

Internal derangement of the joint. This means a dislocated jaw or displaced disk (cushion of cartilage between the head of the jawbone and the skull) or injury to the condyle (the rounded end of the jawbone that articulates with the temporal skull bone).

Degenerative joint disease. This includes osteoarthritis or rheumatoid arthritis in the jaw joint.[72]

You can have one or more of these conditions at the same time.

A recent article in the *Journal of Headache and Pain* makes the point that this can be a difficult diagnostic dilemma.

"The complicated treatment of TMD requires specific knowledge and exercises to strengthen some groups of muscles and weaken others, occlusal splint therapy, massage, and pharmacotherapy. Although the treatment seems difficult, most of the patients searching for help due to TMD assess that the treatment is successful, although an accurate

---

71   "Temporomandibular Disorder (TMD)," hopkinsmedicine.org (Johns Hopkins Medicine, August 8, 2021), https://www.hopkinsmedicine.org/health/conditions-and-diseases/temporomandibular-disorder-tmd#:~:text=Temporomandibular%20disorders%20(TMD)%20are%20disorders,may%20result%20in%20temporomandibular%20disorder.

72   Ibid.

diagnosis needs to be made to start the proper protocol of treatment," the authors observe.[73] People use the "TMJ" term to refer to conditions and diseases of the joint. Some use the abbreviation "TMD" or temporomandibular dysfunction.

The Mayo Clinic reports that TMD has become very common. The US has over three million cases per year, very treatable by a medical professional, and can be self-diagnosable. Lab tests or imaging may not be needed, and in the medium term, it can resolve within months.[74]

I would say that about 25 percent of my adult patients have some sort of signs and symptoms of a temporomandibular dysfunction or disharmony. And less than 0.5 percent do anything about it.

Traditionally, decompression offers a proven approach to try to get some sort of feedback to tell the body, *Hey, stop doing what you're doing and stop loading the joint. Stop putting pressure in that area.* Relax it and try to restore the harmony.

We see symptoms in our patients with worn teeth from nighttime gnashing, grinding, and sliding, and improper breathing. Most have no idea they're actually doing it, a silent sign that there's something going on with the jaw joint because it should be relaxed and calm. Sleep produces periods of parasympathetic activities, mostly "rest and digest" conditions.

The *parasympathetic* nervous system (PNS) predominates in quiet "rest and digest" conditions while the sympathetic nervous system drives the "fight or flight" response in stressful situations. The PNS conserves energy to be used later to regulate bodily functions like digestion and urination when you're sleeping, but people become more hyperactive at night for a reason.

Stress, medicines, or poor sleep can set off the *sympathetic* nervous system, kicking in the *fight or flight* reaction.

---

73   Ibid.

74   "TMJ Disorders," mayoclinic.org (Mayo Foundation for Medical Education and Research, December 28, 2018), https://www.mayoclinic.org/diseases-conditions/tmj/diagnosis-treatment/drc-20350945.

But back to the jaw joint. People fracture their teeth. We see people with virgin teeth that just fracture the cusps or fracture the teeth vertically, where they have loaded their teeth with so much pressure that it causes breakage. We see that all the time.

The wears, the signs, the cracks, and the fractures cannot all be attributed to the jaw joint because we routinely chew and function every day. These could represent cumulative effects. Hot and cold thermal cycling on our teeth can put internal stresses on our teeth, but I generally look for the jaw being overloaded because of bruxing, clenching, or grinding.

So if people say they have vague issues, we investigate a little bit differently and look for signs of sleep disorders. In 2017, the House of Delegates for the American Dental Association issued a position paper that basically says that "dentists can and do play an essential role in the multidisciplinary care of patients with certain sleep-related breathing disorders and are well positioned to identify patients at greater risk. And therefore best treated through a collaborative model." We've been tasked by the American Dental Association to screen patients for sleep disorders.

THE ROLE OF DENTISTRY IN THE TREATMENT OF SLEEP-RELATED BREATHING DISORDERS (SRBD)

Excerpts as adopted by American Dental Association 2017 House of Delegates[75]

- Dentists are encouraged to screen patients for SRBD as part of a comprehensive medical and dental history to recognize symptoms such as daytime sleepiness, choking, snoring, or witnessed apneas and an evaluation for risk factors such as obesity, retrognathia, or hypertension. If the risk for SRBD is determined, these patients should be referred, as needed, to the appropriate physicians for proper diagnosis.

---

75   "TMJ Disorders," mayoclinic.org (Mayo Foundation for Medical Education and Research, December 28, 2018), https://www.mayoclinic.org/diseases-conditions/tmj/diagnosis-treatment/drc-20350945.

- In children, screening through history and clinical examination may identify signs and symptoms of deficient growth and development, or other risk factors that may lead to airway issues. If risk for SRBD is determined, intervention through medical/dental referral or evidenced-based treatment may be appropriate to help treat the SRBD and/or develop an optimal physiologic airway and breathing pattern.

- Oral appliance therapy is an appropriate treatment for mild and moderate sleep apnea, and for severe sleep apnea when the patient does not tolerate a CPAP. (Note: Continuous positive airway pressure—or CPAP—therapy is a common treatment for obstructive sleep apnea. A CPAP machine uses a hose connected to a mask or nosepiece to deliver constant and steady air pressure to help you breathe while you sleep.)

- When oral appliance therapy is prescribed by a physician through written or electronic order for an adult patient with obstructive sleep apnea, a dentist should evaluate the patient for the appropriateness of fabricating a suitable oral appliance. If deemed appropriate, a dentist should fabricate an oral appliance.

- Dentists should maintain regular communications with the patient's referring physician and other healthcare providers to the patient's treatment progress and any recommended follow-up treatment.

Source: American Dental Association[76]

When I screen a patient, and even when I do an annual or semi-annual exam, I will ask questions about their sleep habits. (I learned a long time ago not to ask a lady if she snores. I ask in an unoffensive and nonthreatening way, *Do you sleep well? Do you find that you're well rested?*

---

76 "The Role of Dentistry in the Treatment of Sleep Related Breathing," www.ada.org (American Dental Association, 2017), https://www.ada.org/-/media/project/ada-organization/ada/ada-org/files/resources/research/the-role-of-dentistry-in-sleep-related-breathing-disorders.pdf.

And depending on their honesty, they'll say yes, or no. A lot of people have sleep disorders, and they are not even aware of it. There are screening tests we can do like the Epworth Sleepiness Scale and STOP-BANG questionnaires, and we can do a visual inspection of their soft palette, uvula, and tongue, and can look at that airway space with the mouth open. We use a score on that called a Mallampati score, a simple test that can be a good predictor of obstructive sleep apnea.

Solutions for TMD

Among the solutions created by dentists has been the fabrication of night guards. Many different variations of the types of these devices can be created: a top night guard, lower night guard, and night guards that just fit on the front of your teeth to separate the back teeth from crunching or grinding. It depends on the decade or the era. Is it an upper or lower? We don't necessarily have a perfect handle on what the generic optimal night guard looks like because it's very individualized.

WE DON'T NECESSARILY HAVE A GENERIC OPTIMAL NIGHT GUARD BECAUSE IT'S VERY INDIVIDUALIZED.

There are acute TMD issues, and there are chronic ones.

There could be one from trauma, from a fall, an accident or car crash, or when you slam your teeth together, suddenly. With acute events, the patient can open wide, yawn, and hear a pop, and the muscles that hold the joint in place and the ligaments may go into a spasm, and become dislocated.

We could also have trauma resulting from difficult dental interventions such as wisdom teeth extractions, fillings or crowns, or prolonged procedures. We deal with such acute issues through rest and ice and limiting those motions and maybe general massages, neural therapy, or lasers. After a while, we prescribe heat, or nonsteroidal anti-inflammatories. If severely acute, we may deploy muscle relaxants.

Then there are what we call *chronic problems*, often caused by repetitive trauma such as clenching or grinding, or bruxing.

You can have changes because we change the harmony of your teeth when we put in crowns. Patients can develop a bite that may not be perfectly balanced, and this can develop over the years. These issues can result in headaches or pain that radiates down the neck into the ear. There can be clicking or popping, sounds called crepitus, that comes from that. The jaw can be locked in an open or closed position. It can develop from improper bite alignment. The patient can have a spasm in one direction, and the teeth don't hit normally anymore. There can be swelling.

A silent sign that you clench at night is bone deposition from clenching, a silent sign that you do have a growing problem.

In the lower jaw, behind your lips, and in front of your tongue, tori can develop. Tori are bumps in the mouth made of bone tissue covered by gum tissue. They grow slowly and some people have them without ever noticing them. They often grow over a period of time. In fact, a bone can develop all along the gum line of your teeth where you're developing shelves of bone.

The Most Common Signs and Symptoms of TMD

- Jaw discomfort or soreness (often most prevalent in the morning or late afternoon)

- Headaches

- Pain spreading behind the eyes, in the face, shoulder, neck, and/or back

- Earaches or ringing in the ears (not caused by an infection of the inner ear canal)

- Clicking or popping of the jaw

- Locking of the jaw

- Limited mouth motions

- Clenching or grinding of the teeth

- Dizziness

- Sensitivity of the teeth without the presence of an oral health disease

- Numbness or tingling sensation in the fingers

- A change in the way the upper and lower teeth fit together[77]

SELF-CARE FOR TMJ DISORDERS

LIFESTYLE AND HOME REMEDIES[78]

The following tips may help you reduce symptoms of TMJ disorders:

- Becoming more aware of tension-related habits—clenching your jaw, grinding your teeth, or chewing pencils—will help you reduce their frequency.

- Avoid overuse of jaw muscles. Eat soft foods. Cut food into small pieces. Steer clear of sticky or chewy food. Avoid chewing gum.

- Stretching and massage. Your doctor, dentist, or physical therapist may show you how to do exercises that stretch and strengthen your jaw muscles and how to massage the muscles yourself.

---

77 "Temporomandibular Disorder (TMD)," hopkinsmedicine.org (Johns Hopkins Medicine, August 8, 2021), https://www.hopkinsmedicine.org/health/conditions-and-diseases/temporomandibular-disorder-tmd#:~:text=Temporomandibular%20disorders%20(TMD)%20are%20disorders,may%20result%20in%20temporomandibular%20disorder.

78 "TMJ Disorders," mayoclinic.org (Mayo Foundation for Medical Education and Research, December 28, 2018), https://www.mayoclinic.org/diseases-conditions/tmj/diagnosis-treatment/drc-20350945.

- Heat or cold. Applying warm, moist heat or ice to the side of your face may help alleviate pain.

- Complementary and alternative medicine techniques may help manage the chronic pain often associated with TMJ disorders. Examples include:

Acupuncture. A specialist trained in acupuncture treats chronic pain by inserting hair-thin needles at specific locations on your body.

Relaxation techniques. Consciously slowing your breathing and taking deep, regular breaths can help relax tense muscles, which can reduce pain.

Biofeedback. Electronic devices that monitor the tightness of specific muscles can help you practice effective relaxation techniques.

Breathing and Sleep Issues

If I see a restricted airway in a patient, and they have poor sleep habits, then I refer them to their physician to discuss their sleep habits and sleep patterns and see if any of their systemic issues or pharmaceutical use, could affect sleep. If I can't see the airway clearly, then I question how much resistance is occurring. We cannot tell if a person has sleep apnea without a sleep test. That could be a hospital-based, clinic-based test, or home test. Once we get the result of that, sleep disorders get graded into mild, moderate, or severe, and the physician will make a recommendation. And if it's above a certain threshold, the patient will be prescribed a CPAP machine.

The problem with that is, over a period of time, people become less tolerant of the use of the CPAP device. They stop using it. They cause harm by limiting oxygen to the brain and vital organs. It causes slow havoc to the body system.

Dentists can work in conjunction with the physician to fabricate oral appliances for mild or moderate cases, or in cases where a patient can't or won't tolerate a CPAP machine.

We do notice a correlation between obesity and sleep troubles, which can be clearly measured with the Epworth Sleepiness Scale or STOP-BANG questionnaire, detailing the body mass index, neck size, and gender, and then assigning the patient to a category. And again, it's just a screening tool. But I do think being overweight plays a part in many systemic issues, including sleep apnea or sleep disorders.

I am six feet tall. I weigh about 170 pounds. I've been this weight for many decades, but I do not have a thick neck. I wear a size sixteen neck collar and a size forty-two suit long jacket, pretty normal. I am not a big guy. My waist size for my pants tops out at thirty-three (if I could find them). I don't have a weight problem. But for years I knew I had a growl, and a snore, and a snort, so to speak, in my sleep, as described by my wife. And then I just stopped snoring, the Great End-of-Snoring mystery. Recently, I took a home sleep test, and I have moderate sleep apnea, but I do not fit the stereotypical patient.

So what am I doing about it? Well, I haven't yet made my mandibular advancement appliance, the usual remedy, where it brings the lower jaw forward, which brings the tongue forward and away from the soft palate and the uvula, and it creates less resistance for air to flow through.

You may not have been told this, but nasal breathing is important. A patient's airway with minimal resistance may be a result of becoming a mouth breather at night or during the day, and that changes the posture of your head and neck. It creates cervical strain and facial pain. So by restoring proper nasal breathing, we could bring the chin back, and the head up a little bit, straightening out and putting the proper curves back in the spine, reducing head, neck, and shoulder pain.

We experience less resistance to breathing through our nose than our mouth.

Significant benefits result from breathing through your nose and having cleaner air that passes through. It helps create nitric oxide, which effectively helps reduce the bacterial load coming through your nose, enhancing protection, especially during flu and widespread virus times. Proper nasal breathing and proper nasal health are going to reduce the potential for sleep issues or sleep breathing issues.

> **PROPER NASAL BREATHING AND PROPER NASAL HEALTH ARE GOING TO REDUCE THE POTENTIAL FOR SLEEP ISSUES OR SLEEP BREATHING ISSUES.**

The first way I attacked my problem has been to wear Breathe Right strips across the bridge of my nose, and it opened up my nasal passages, and it made me breathe better, especially at night. I felt better rested, even though I sleep well anyway.

In addition, my ENT physician did the VivAer procedure, using radio frequencies and heat. This opened up my nasal passages, increasing my nasal valve and creating less resistance to breathing through my nose. VivAer nasal airway remodeling represents a new cutting-edge technology that uses radiofrequency energy to remodel/reshape the cartilage of your nose and open the nasal valve without altering the outward look of your nose. My ENT physician noted that I also had a slightly deviated septum. This procedure did not fix that, but this was the least offensive way that I could go through without having a nose-jaw rhinoplasty done, and I wouldn't have to use Breathe Right strips for the rest of my life.

I definitely have an ENT doctor who understands, and who's in tune to sleep and proper nasal breathing, because that's what these doctors do. They work on the nose, the ears, and the throat. And if this does not provide a better resolution to my dilemma, I will make a mandibular appliance, which brings my jaw forward.

Oral Appliances

Mandibular repositioning appliances are used to change the shape of the airway. The Food and Drug Administration has cleared a number of oral appliance devices as safe and effective. These devices may be intended to permanently adjust the patient into a more protrusive position, altering the rest position of the jaw joints.

Oral appliance therapy or mandibular advancement splints are retentive and adjustable. They usually cover both the top and bottom jaws, and by the way, are usually comfortable and minimally invasive. There are several options for these appliances out there.

These devices will cause teeth to shift a little bit and possibly create some discomfort in the jaw joint. But that can be dealt with on a daily basis. If the patient holds their jaw forward all night long, the muscles are not used to the jaw being there. They get tight. Not that they're going to cause chronic TMJ issues, but patients may wake up where the jaw has become stiff, and their teeth don't line up. They may have to move the jaw around to get them back to where they have to go. That's a disadvantage of wearing one of these things. Over time, the teeth may shift in position a little bit. It can happen to anyone.

Many dentists have been trained in sleep medicine to make these devices. And they're FDA-approved. The TMJ and the sleep problem can present a challenge because dentists have been trained for years to respond to a patient with a jaw joint problem by making a mouth guard to decompress the joint. Night guards can be a double-edged sword. If the patient has a sleep issue overlapping the TMJ disorder, it can actually make things worse. That's why we screen for sleep if they have TMJ issues because of the interconnection between the two.

Some people can get relief from a craniosacral massage. This light massage to the head, upper neck, and spine can release tensions associated with TMJ dysfunction and improve total well-being.

VITAL BODY PROCESSES OCCUR DURING SLEEP[79]

During sleep, your body is busy.

- Repairing tissues.
- Fighting off infections.
- Forming memories of experiences that occurred during the day.

If you do not get adequate sleep, you could experience health effects such as

- Disruption of the insulin/blood glucose system, promoting insulin resistance.
- Increased appetite, resulting in overeating and weight gain.
- Impaired mental functioning.

Sleep loss can also weaken the immune system by

- Reducing the proper function of cells that attack cancer cells and viruses.
- Increasing the inflammatory response, which increases the risk for cardiovascular and metabolic disorders such as diabetes.
- Reducing the production of antibodies, thereby increasing the risk of infection.

---

79   "Vital Body Processes Occur during Sleep," cdc.gov (Centers for Disease Control and Prevention, April 1, 2020), https://www.cdc.gov/niosh/emres/longhourstraining/vital.html.

I would say at least half of my patients will go for the referral for a sleep issue if they have TMJ issues because they're not breathing properly. About half of those folks do not breathe properly through their nose, and the other half have obstructive sleep issues. It may not be nasally related, but they have some issue. Those patients are not sleeping well. TMJ, facial pain, and sleep issues go hand in hand.

When confronted with difficult diagnostic dilemmas like TMJ disorder, we all have to put on a Sherlock Holmes outfit.

In 2019, the National Academy of Medicine (NAM) undertook its first study of temporomandibular disorders. The effort resulted in a landmark report published in March 2020 titled "Temporomandibular Disorders: From Research Discoveries to Clinical Treatment." It examines the entire spectrum of TMJ disorders or TMD research, education and training, diagnosis and assessment, clinical management and treatment, comorbidities, treatment efficacy, models of care, insurance practices, clinical translation, and other issues.[80]

We hope this study will lead to a healthcare system better informed by evidence and better equipped to address the complexity of patients with TMD and coexisting medical conditions with an individualized, patient-centered, whole-person approach. I respond very well to empirical evidence, and I wish for a lot more of that.

But either way, the first responder to TMJ will likely be the dentist's office.

Stress

If I encounter a diagnostic situation where I become convinced that life stress causes my patient's issue, I suggest a visit to their primary

---

80   "TMJ Disorders: From Research Discoveries to Clinical Treatment (2020)," tmj.org (The TMJ Association, June 7, 2021), https://tmj.org/hope-in-research/landmark-studies/national-academy-of-medicine/.

care physician. It could involve medicines or metabolic issues. It could be hormonal. That's another problem that disrupts sleep.

I like the new wearable technologies available to score your sleep and readiness to meet the day. The Oura Ring and Apple Watch take the guesswork out of the impact of good sleep on your health and keep an eye on your vital functions. Devices like these monitor heart rate, workouts, sleep, restorative time, oxygen saturation, heart rate variability, body temperature, and readiness for the day. The Oura Ring can also be a helpful tool for spotting changes in your entire body during your menstrual cycle by delivering accurate, personalized resting heart rate, heart rate variability (HRV), respiratory rate, sleep, and body temperature trends.

> **I LIKE WEARABLE TECHNOLOGIES TO SCORE YOUR SLEEP AND READINESS TO MEET THE DAY; THEY TAKE THE GUESSWORK OUT OF THE IMPACT OF GOOD SLEEP AND KEEP AN EYE ON YOUR VITAL FUNCTIONS.**

The Oura Ring keeps track of how much time is spent in each sleep stage, and more. That's pretty useful. You can self-monitor between your physician visits or use that to self-monitor before and after using a dental device or a CPAP machine.

The Apple Watch also monitors this data, watching for arrhythmias like A-fib. Very important, because cardiovascular issues can arise from poor-quality sleep.

Readiness gives you a key Oura score, designed for you and only you, that may help you discover what works for your body and lifestyle. Readiness develops a holistic picture of your health—considering your recent activity, sleep patterns, and direct body signals (like resting heart rate, heart rate variability, and body temperature) that can signify if your body is under strain.

I think it would be wonderful as a biologic dentist to have this information on all my patients at the point of care.

Your readiness score ranges from 0–100 and tells you at-a-glance if you are ready to face greater challenges or if you need some recovery and rest:

- 85 or higher: Optimal, you're ready for action!

- 70–84: Good, you've recovered well enough.

- Under 70: Pay attention, you're not fully recovered.[81]

Who would have thought that at this stage of our life, a ring would team up with a watch or cell phone to help us take better care of ourselves? How great is that!

So, you can recover from TMJ, just as Muhammad Ali recovered from his broken jaw.

Sports Illustrated summed it up. "If you have counted out Muhammad Ali as the next heavyweight champion of the entire universe, forget it.

"In the next couple of years, he will knock out Ken Norton in four rounds, Joe Frazier in six and win his championship back from George Foreman by a technical knockout in thirteen."[82]

In the next chapter, we will recall another legend; this one involves the Tooth Fairy tale where a mouse knocked out the king's teeth.

81   "Your Oura Readiness Score," ouraring.com (Oura Health, September 2, 2020), https://ouraring. com/blog/readiness-score/.

82   Tex Maule, "The Mouth That Nearly Roared," si.com (*Sports Illustrated*, September 24, 2015), https:// www.si.com/boxing/2015/09/24/muhammad-ali-broken-jaw.

CHAPTER 7:

SLEEP AND BIOLOGIC DENTAL CARE FOR KIDS

The mouse turns out to be a fairy who frees the queen and knocks out the king's teeth.

Biologic dentistry uniquely approaches oral care for children and young adults. We do not pull every wisdom tooth, we do not overuse fluoride, focusing on diet and oral care instead, and we do not use amalgam fillings. We do not automatically recommend metal braces, and if braces are needed, we like the new clear aligners a lot. We bring to the dental chair all of our advanced tools such as lasers and ozone and mercury-free dentistry.

SO I MAKE SURE THAT CHILDREN CAN BREATHE PROPERLY.

Children must sleep soundly because it affects their ability to function well in school. If a child does not sleep well, a lot of things can go wrong from bed-wetting to acting out, and poor performance in school because they are half asleep and their attentiveness falters.

So I make sure that children can breathe properly. I consider their diet and allergies, sensitivities, and especially, their oral anatomy.

In early infancy, the baby needs to be able to swallow properly because teeth have not yet arrived. The tongue needs to sit up against the palate and apply a force while the face grows. Because most of our face grows within the first few years of our life, proper swallowing needs to be established almost immediately. And when that happens, our tongue can help guide bone formation. If the midface and lower face get wide enough, then primary teeth come in the right spot, they're not crowded, and a crossbite does not develop.

We seek the optimal scenario for the tongue and teeth to fit harmoniously. We continue on with a nice diet, a dense diet that also promotes the proper growth of the skeletal system and our facial system. When we do that, and our tongue fits properly against our palate, our lips are sealed because our teeth fit in the right spot. Our lips can close over our teeth. They're not bucked out.

Then we can start breathing smoothly through our nose, and we train ourselves to be nasal breathers. That creates mid-facial width and promotes good, long-term, proper breathing.

Tongue-Tie

The mouth and bone structure need to be the right width in order for the tongue to fit properly.

And if the tongue fits in the mouth properly, then swallowing will be appropriate. Breathing, chewing, and swallowing will all work together properly.

Structurally, you can be born with your tongue kind of tied to the lower part of your mouth. We call that tongue-tie, an easier-to-remember name for ankyloglossia. Tongue-tie can contribute to poor swallowing, poor tongue posture, flinching, grinding of the teeth, jaw problems, jaw pain, poor sleep, speech issues, or poor cranial sacral flow. Sacral flow is your brain clearing out your toxins. We previously reviewed that involvement with the glial system.

So the tongue-tie needs to be identified early on. A fair number of adults have not pursued a correction and are partially tongue-tied. Perhaps they do not realize it.

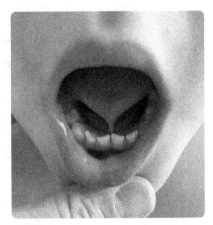

Infant and Pediatric Frenectomies

In the past, the frenectomy procedure was perhaps the most popular soft tissue operation in younger patients. Many labial and lingual frenum (tongue and lip ties) were snipped by a midwife, family doctor, or dental surgeon. Hospital nursery staff often are the first to notice that a newborn does not eat well. These nurses are vigilant for tongue-ties. The overall awareness and treatment of tongue and lip ties, especially in breastfeeding infants, has increased over recent years, much due to the great work of lactation consultants. The lactation nurses are all over that, championing the baby-mother bond through breastfeeding. Frenectomies are routinely performed on infants to improve breastfeeding outcomes.

Traditionally, we could diagnose tongue-ties by appearance alone; newer research advocates for a functional assessment to determine any deleterious effect on breastfeeding. Before any surgical intervention for difficulties related to breastfeeding, we always refer to a certified lactation consultant.

THE CLEVELAND CLINIC: WHAT IS THE PURPOSE OF A FRENECTOMY?

There are many reasons why you or your child might need a frenectomy. This procedure can correct a frenum that's causing:

- A lip tie, which limits lip movement
- A tongue-tie, which limits your tongue's range of motion
- Diastema (a gap between your teeth), which may be cosmetically displeasing to some people
- Gum recession, which can lead to gingivitis, cavities, and mobility
- Pain, swelling, or tenderness with brushing or oral care[83]

Sometimes a frenum can be so tight that it pulls the gums away from the teeth. A frenectomy frees the band of connective tissue, reducing the risk of gaps, gum recession, and other oral health problems.

The soft tissue laser can safely and efficiently release frenectomies with predictable and repeatable tissue response. The precise cutting, and clear and bloodless operating field, make the laser a good choice for frenectomy procedures. Laser oral surgery also provides less wound contraction and reduced scarring or fibrosis compared to scalpel incisions.

FRENECTOMY SURGERY OFFERS SEVERAL BENEFITS:

- Solves breastfeeding problems in infants
- Improves speech problems caused by tongue-tie
- Reduces the risk of tooth decay, gum disease, and other oral health problems
- Enhances the appearance of the smile by eliminating gaps

---

83   "Frenectomy: What It Is, Procedure & Recovery," https://my.clevelandclinic.org/ (Cleveland Clinic, April 11, 2022), https://my.clevelandclinic.org/health/treatments/22714-frenectomy#:~:text=A%20 frenectomy%20is%20an%20oral,a%20wide%20range%20of%20benefits.

Traditionally, there have been two ways to do it. There has been the traditional way with scissors or the scalpel after anesthesia.

For a newborn, some doctors use scissors to cut and release it. But that's just the initial release. The fascia must also be released, the tissue between the tongue and the bone behind the front lower teeth. It's just not a single guitar string. There are multiple bands in there. Then typically, we suture that up.

Often, with anesthesia, we deploy the Erbium-YAG laser to release the tissue.

Nd:YAG lasers were the first types of true pulsed lasers developed exclusively for dental use beginning in 1990. I also use the laser for the treatment of snoring (NightLase), periodontal therapy, and red light therapy (photo-biomodulation). It's a very big tool in my tool chest.

Deviated Septum

As the child grows older, nasal breathing is important. Young people rarely have had a deviated septum through trauma. But developmentally, a child can have a deviated septum, which could affect nasal breathing, making the child more of an oral mouth breather. This concerns us because it can collapse the arch of your teeth and create malocclusion, crowding, or buck teeth. And then you can't get a good lip seal.

An Alternate Tooth Fairy Legend

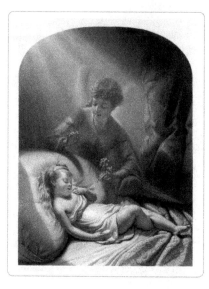

European history offers several Tooth Fairy legends. There was an old British custom of giving *fairy coins* to servant girls while they slept, but this did not involve teeth.

Irish folk tradition includes fairy *changelings*, so it's possible that a tooth placed near a sleeping child could serve to fool a malevolent spirit.

There's also a Venetian version of the Italian Befana, who acts as Santa Claus who gives presents or a coin to a child who has lost a tooth.

And in late-nineteenth-century France, one tradition has the Virgin Mary exchanging a coin or presents for a tooth left under a child's pillow.

But the closest parallel to the American Tooth Fairy may be an eighteenth-century French fairy tale *La Bonne Petite Souris*. In the story, a good queen, imprisoned by a bad king, enlists a mouse for help out of her predicament. The mouse turns out to be a fairy who frees the queen and knocks out the king's teeth. The fairy-mouse then hides the teeth under the king's pillow, before eventually having him assassinated. A happy children's tale for sure![84]

---

84   Kristina Killgrove, "Where Did the Tooth Fairy Come From?," forbes.com (*Forbes*, September 14, 2016), https://www.forbes.com/sites/kristinakillgrove/2016/09/14/where-did-the-tooth-fairy-come-from/?sh=4ebd8ade59d4.

Articulation Issues

About breastfeeding, if the baby latches on, then we're thriving. After babies make it through to age two with no issues, I begin to assess for proper speech all the way to age five.

I make sure to guide parents to recognize articulation issues. I want to hear a child speak crisply and cleanly, and phonetically. I want to hear it. All of my children have gone through speech and articulation therapy to crisp up their sounds. I'm not sure why all of my children needed it, but there were problems. I am acutely aware of a child with a lisp, a hiss, or something just not right. Then I have an in-depth discussion with the parents.

Parents usually realize pretty early that their child does not have the development needed at that particular age. I guide them to speech pathologists.

I think it's a great thing that we recognize that early on. Because, for example, in many US communities, acceptance into a school-based special needs program or county-based program is very difficult. Kids have to be quite unintelligible to get help from a public school.

Stanford Medicine Newborn Nursery urges parents and dentists to work directly with the speech pathologist to evaluate the child orally to make sure that they do not have a structural dental mouth issue that could be causing them not to be able to articulate their words, breathe properly, or swallow properly.[85]

Tonsils or Enlarged Tongue

Why do children have tonsillitis? It could be viruses or bacteria. Perhaps it's food allergies or sensitivities. Why are we more sensitive

---

85   "What Is Frenectomy?," https://med.stanford.edu/ (Stanford Medicine), accessed February 7, 2023, https://med.stanford.edu/newborns/professional-education/frenotomy.html.

to food or the environment? Genetics? The patient's ear, nose, and throat specialist will assess the tonsils and adenoids to see if they need to come out.

We frequently encounter an enlarged tongue. People can have macroglossia for a reason, a disorder characterized by a tongue that is large in proportion to other structures in the mouth. In the congenital type of the disorder, protrusion of the tongue from the mouth may interfere with the feeding of the infant. The culprit can sometimes be some sort of swelling or chronic allergies if they cause chronic postnasal drip, or runny nose, especially at night. Food sensitivities can potentially cause an enlargement of the tongue. These patients become mouth breathers because their nose isn't behaving properly.

Enlargement of the tongue can decrease proper sleep. If our tonsils are enlarged, it creates more of an open mouth. An open-mouth breather brings the jaw forward and the neck stretched forward to breathe easier. It can generate a posture problem, which can cause facial and neck pain.

So all of those oral structures and deficiencies in their proper function can create issues that can lead to poor sleep or poor breathing.

Many of the dental experiences our children have also occur in adulthood, and an awful lot has to do with sleep, and Shakespeare.

SLEEP AND BIOLOGIC DENTAL CARE FOR ADULTS FOR BETTER SLEEP AND BETTER BREATHING

To sleep—perchance to dream. Ay, there's the rub!

These memorable words are from Shakespeare's famous "To be or not to be" soliloquy in Act 3 Scene 1 of the 1602 play *Hamlet*, when Prince Hamlet said, "To sleep; perchance to dream: ay there's the rub."[86]

Hamlet's message was not really about sleep but about contemplating life or the end of life to solve a vexing problem.

I remember when playing baseball as a kid, if a player got hit hard with a ball, the coach would yell, "Rub it hard." That didn't really take the pain away, but it was something. We actually believed that it would help the situation. (Well-intentioned coaching, but not-so-great in pain relief.)

---

86   William Shakespeare, *Hamlet*, Act 3 Scene 1, quoted in, "To Sleep Perchance to Dream, Meaning & Context," No Sweat Shakespeare, accessed September 30, 2022, https://nosweatshakespeare. com/quotes/famous/to-sleep-perchance-to-dream/.

"Rub" in this sense means drawback or impediment, the most significant issue or problem in a situation. And for sixty million Americans, that's a great symbol of the problem of improper sleep. If we cannot sleep properly, everything else doesn't work right.

There's the rub.

Besides the stress of not getting a good night's sleep, sleep disorders can have a lasting impact on health and well-being. It's essential to seek treatment. A doctor may recommend lifestyle changes, medications, or a sleep study for those suffering from sleep disorders.

Sleep Deprivation Effects

Johns Hopkins Medicine notes that lack of sleep deserves our attention and a doctor's help. "Not getting enough sleep—due to insomnia or a sleep disorder such as obstructive sleep apnea, or simply because you're keeping late hours—can affect your mood, memory, and health in far-reaching and surprising ways," says Johns Hopkins sleep researcher Patrick Finan, PhD. Sleep deprivation can also affect your judgment, so you don't notice its effects.[87]

And there's more to this rub.

EFFECTS OF SLEEP DEPRIVATION

- 6,000 fatal car crashes are caused by drowsy driving each year.

- One in twenty-five adults has fallen asleep at the wheel in the past month.

- 33 percent increase in dementia risk.

- Can age your brain three to five years.

---

87   "The Effects of Sleep Deprivation," hopkinsmedicine.org (John Hopkins Medicine, October 21, 2021), https://www.hopkinsmedicine.org/health/wellness-and-prevention/the-effects-of-sleep-deprivation.

- 48 percent increase in developing heart disease.

- Three times more likely to catch a cold.

- 36 percent increase in risk for colorectal cancer.

- Three times the risk for type 2 diabetes.

- 50 percent risk of obesity if you get less than five hours of sleep a night.[88]

So, as we contemplate this rub, we see that sleep disorders can be more than an irritation, or a snoring issue; these disorders can make a significant impact on the quality of your life.

Millions of Americans suffer from sporadic poor sleep that can be managed through stress reduction, diet, and natural sleep aids. However, several types of sleep conditions require clinical care by a physician or other healthcare professional. These sleep conditions include insomnia, sleepwalking, sleep apnea, narcolepsy, and restless legs syndrome.

Adult humans need to sleep between seven and nine hours to feel rested. Lack of sleep can be associated with bad sleeping habits or health issues such as anxiety, depression, persistent pain, or cancer. Sleep, an active state that filters external inputs, provides a natural process that enables us to recover from our energy expenditure during wakefulness. It also contributes to mood maintenance, immune system recovery, brain and muscle regeneration, and memory consolidation.

Sleep follows an (approximately) twenty-four-hour cycle under light and environmental cues.

The Journal of Oral Rehabilitation reports in a 2020 article, "The Face of Dental Sleep Medicine in the 21st Century," that during sleep, the cortex is relatively quiet, except during specific phases of arousal

---

88   "Sleep Conditions," hopkinsmedicine.org (Johns Hopkins Medicine), accessed February 7, 2023, https://www.hopkinsmedicine.org/health/wellness-and-prevention/sleep-conditions.

that naturally occur every twenty to forty seconds. These arousals are cyclic physiological phenomena that appear to preserve homeostasis and survival.

"Arousals are characterized by three- to ten-second increases in, amongst others: heart rate; autonomic nervous system, brain and muscle activities; and body temperature. Their main function is to preserve sleep stability or to trigger a full awakening that can be associated with a fight or flight survival reaction," the authors observe.[89]

Pain during sleep, like any sensory input such as sound, will trigger arousals, and when needed, full awakenings to assure body protection, the authors note.

Reciprocally, sleep also influences pain. For example, three to four nights of experimental sleep deprivation may trigger mood alteration and initiate pain complaints in healthy subjects.

Two Types of Sleep

There are two major types of sleep that your body cycles through to get a good night's rest: non-rapid eye movement sleep and rapid eye movement, or REM, sleep.

While non-REM sleep assists in hormone regulation and protein synthesis during muscle recovery, REM sleep helps with emotional processing and boosting good mental health. Rapid eye movement sleep comes at the end of the night, the sleep stage most likely to be missed if one isn't getting enough sleep.

Harvard Medical School reports that low-quality sleep and sleep deprivation also negatively impact mood, which has consequences for learning.

---

89   F. Lobbezoo, G.J. Lavigne, T. Kato, F.R. de Almeida, G. Aarab, "The Face of Dental Sleep Medicine in the 21st Century," *Journal of Oral Rehabilitation* (August 29, 2020), https://www.ncbi.nlm.nih.gov/pmc/articles/PMC7754359.

"Alterations in mood affect our ability to acquire new information and subsequently to remember that information. Although chronic sleep deprivation affects different individuals in a variety of ways (and the effects are not entirely known), it is clear that a good night's rest has a strong impact on learning and memory."[90]

As the night goes on, the REM proportion of your sleep cycle gets longer and longer, which explains why you tend to wake up remembering the final dream of the sleep period. Each sleep cycle does not stand alone, and all of them are required in order to get a good night's sleep.[91]

The benefits of getting good sleep can go beyond daily performance and can, in some cases, prevent long-term problems. Everything you experience files away into your long-term memory during sleep, and when your brain does this filing, it also assigns the proper emotional response to each memory.

The Role of the Dentist in Sleep Disorders[92]

Suggested strategies for the management of oro-facial pain and sleep interaction by dentists.

- Assess whether comorbidities like lousy life habits, mood alteration, bruxism, or adverse oral habits are contributing to the oro-facial pain condition.

- Suggest improvements in sleep hygiene, relaxation therapy, yoga, etc.

---

90   "Sleep, Learning, and Memory," https://healthysleep.med.harvard.edu/healthy/ (Harvard Medical School, December 18, 2007), https://healthysleep.med.harvard.edu/healthy/matters/benefits-of-sleep/learning-memory.

91   Ibid.

92   Frank Lobbezoo et al., "The Face of Dental Sleep Medicine in the 21st Century," https://pubmed.ncbi.nlm.nih.gov/ (U.S. National Library of Medicine, August 29, 2020), https://pubmed.ncbi.nlm.nih.gov/32799330/.

- Refer to a psychologist or physical therapist when indicated.

- Confirm the role of other sleep disorders by a sleep physician who may conduct sleep testing/recording. Except for sleep bruxism without sleep comorbidities, the diagnosis and management of sleep disorders, such as insomnia, apnea, periodic limb movement, and REM behavior disorders, are done by sleep physicians.

- Consider, after diagnosis of sleep disorders, an occlusal splint if no obstructive sleep apnea is present, or a mandibular advancement device if headache and/or sleep-breathing issues are present.

- Prescribe non-steroidal analgesics and muscle relaxants as a management option for the short term. Avoid benzodiazepines or opioids if sleep-disordered breathing, RERA (respiratory effort-related arousal), or apnea are suspected. RERA is an event characterized by increasing respiratory effort for ten seconds or longer leading to an arousal from sleep but one that does not fulfill the criteria for a hypopnea or apnea.

- Physicians may prescribe sleeping pills or other more powerful medication to improve the deleterious pain and sleep interaction.

With the exception of sleep bruxism without sleep comorbidities, the diagnosis and management of sleep disorders, such as insomnia, apnea, periodic limb movement, and REM behavior disorders, are done by sleep physicians.

I carefully evaluate my patients. I look at their oral structures and their tone. We will have a thoughtful discussion about it. The American Dental Association says dentists should be screening their patients for sleep apnea and should be the professionals who make oral appliances.

While most sleep disorders should be diagnosed and treated by medical doctors, it becomes increasingly clear that some disorders have important diagnostic and/or management links to the dental domain, hence the emergence of the discipline "dental sleep medicine" in dentistry.

We define dental sleep medicine as the study of the oral and maxillofacial causes and consequences of sleep-related problems.

Over twenty years ago, the literature lit up with articles about dental involvement in the diagnosis and treatment of sleep disorders. Several common sleep disorders of interest to dentists were described, namely sleep-related oro-facial pain, oro-facial movement disorders, breathing disorders, oral moistening disorders, and gastro-esophageal reflux, all of which require the attention of dentists.[93]

Dental sleep medicine has taken shape in the twenty-first century, benefiting all patients suffering from dental sleep disorders.

KEY POINTS

Sleep-related breathing disorders comprise a variety of diagnoses, including simple snoring, hypopnea, upper airway resistance syndrome, central sleep apnea, and obstructive sleep apnea (OSA). OSA is the most prevalent form of sleep apnea, accounting for over 80 percent of sleep-disordered breathing cases in the US.

---

93   Ibid.

Sleep Apnea

Eighteen million people.

That's close to the total population of New York State if we black out New York Mets fans.

That's how many Americans have sleep apnea, according to the National Sleep Foundation. The condition causes repeated breathing interruptions throughout the night; the pauses can last from a few seconds to minutes and may occur thirty or more times per hour. *WebMD* writer Jodi Helmer notes that "These pauses happen because the muscles in the back of the throat are flaccid, the tongue too large, or the jaw too small, causing airway obstructions."[94]

There are also a lot more clues to point to a sleep disorder. That's why we call it a difficult diagnostic dilemma. We have to sort things out a bit.

Other clues that the patient may have a sleep disturbance, or a sleep disorder include:

- Tooth wear, which can be severe in patients with sleep bruxism (grinding), and patients with obstructive sleep apnea (OSA)

- Temporomandibular disorder (TMD)

- Gastro-esophageal reflux

- Morning headache and jaw symptoms often associated with primary snoring, OSA, and primary insomnias

- Stress

- Smoking

- Alcohol

---

94   Jodi Helmer, WebMD, "The Link Between Sleep Apnea and Your Dentist," https://www.webmd.com/oral-health/features/link-sleep-apnea-dentist, accessed October 3, 2022.

- Chronic facial pain

- Caffeine

- Sleep-related breathing disorders that comprise a variety of diagnoses

- Simple snoring

- Hypopnea (ten seconds or more of shallow breathing in which a person's airflow drops by at least 30 percent)

- Upper airway resistance syndrome

- Central sleep apnea (a disorder in which someone's breathing repeatedly stops and starts during sleep)

- Obstructive sleep apnea

The WebMD post titled "The Link between Sleep Apnea and Your Dentist," describes the first sign of sleep apnea as tooth grinding (also called bruxism). That's one of the first things I look for, worn tooth surfaces, a sign that a patient grinds their teeth. Grinding can cause tooth wear and breakage, as well as inflamed and receding gums. A spike in cavities can also be a sign of grinding because the force damages teeth, making them susceptible to cavity-causing bacteria.

At night while sleeping, your jaw becomes tense, and you're grinding your teeth. This sends a clear message to your brain to wake up and take a breath. Other oral health signs of sleep apnea include a tongue with scalloped edges, a small jaw, or redness in the throat caused by acute snoring.

Gasping for breath causes people to wake up repeatedly, greatly reducing sleep quality. It causes fatigue. Sleep apnea precipitates a higher risk of obesity, high blood pressure, heart disease, and diabetes.

Obstructive sleep apnea, the most prevalent form of sleep apnea, accounts for over 80 percent of sleep-disordered breathing cases in the US. The American Dental Association characterizes OSA as a "recurrent narrowing or collapse of the upper airway during sleep, resulting in partial or complete cessation of airflow despite the continued respiratory effort."[95]

When taking patient health histories and conducting oral clinical examinations, we screen patients for OSA-related risk factors or common presenting features, such as:

- Large tongue or tonsils.

- Mandibular retrognathia (abnormal placement of the mandible) or micrognathia (an abnormally small mandible).

- Large neck circumference.

- Nocturnal choking or gasping.

- Obesity.

- Loud or irregular snoring.

- Breathing pauses during sleep (if reported by bed partner).

I always refer patients who have these symptoms to a primary care physician or sleep medicine specialist for further evaluation.

Various treatment options include the use of positive airway pressure (CPAP) therapy. A CPAP machine uses a hose connected to a mask or nosepiece to deliver constant and steady air pressure to help you breathe while you sleep.

Common problems with CPAP include a leaky mask, trouble falling asleep, feeling claustrophobic, a stuffy nose, and a dry mouth. But if a CPAP mask or machine doesn't work for you, we have other

---

95   "Sleep Apnea—Obstructive," ada.org (American Dental Association, January 9, 2023), https://www.ada. org/resources/research/science-and-research-institute/oral-health-topics/sleep-apnea-obstructive.

options. Most CPAP masks can be adjusted to help make them more comfortable, but oral appliance therapy may be an option for patients with mild to moderate apnea, an alternative to CPAP for sleep apnea patients who cannot tolerate all the necessary apparatus at night. We create custom oral appliances in our practice, but there are retail versions on the market, often called *snoring appliance* or a *mouthpiece for sleep apnea*. In my opinion, an over-the-counter night guard might not correct the problem by itself and may even make sleep apnea worse.

A sleep oral appliance can help with better breathing during sleep. It's noninvasive and less obtrusive than a CPAP machine. You might have to wear an oral appliance during the day or at night or both, if the treatment included TMJ issues. But most often, we suggest an evening wearable, where it's like a splint to move the lower jaw forward a little bit to bring your tongue out of the way, increasing the volume of the airway.

Snoring and NightLase

Your sleep doctor can evaluate whether the dental treatments are working or not. For snoring, I have found great success with NightLase.

Fotona's NightLase therapy is a noninvasive, patient-friendly laser treatment for increasing the quality of a patient's sleep. NightLase reduces the effects of sleep apnea and decreases the amplitude of snoring by means of a gentle, laser-induced tightening effect caused by the contraction of collagen in the oral mucosa tissue.

So the NightLase uses both energy frequencies of the Fotona Lightwalker. I recently had a patient have a sleep test, and the result was a diagnosis of mild sleep apnea. Then she had to make some decisions. If her diagnosis were severe sleep apnea, she would be hooking up to a CPAP machine at night for sure. But for mild or moderate apnea, her options became the CPAP adventure, maybe a mandibular advancement appliance, or in a mild case, the NightLase procedure, basically a noninvasive treatment in which laser lights are used to heat the tissues to tighten them, leading to a more open airway. Breathing becomes easier, which can result in little or no snoring at all.

Research has shown that NightLase reduces and attenuates snoring and provides an effective, noninvasive way to lessen the effects of sleep apnea. A two-step procedure, there's a preheating, and then the laser treatment. It takes about forty-five minutes to complete. There's no anesthesia. Afterward, you have a little bit of a dry mouth. It's done consecutively, typically on four different occasions, three weeks apart, with some touch-up treatments every six to twelve months, and possibly a follow-up sleep test to measure success.

I tell my patients that NightLase is like getting your hair dyed or teeth whitened; it's not hard and not a forever thing. Patients find NightLase to be a highly comfortable and satisfying solution. It requires no device to be worn during sleep and involves no chemical treatment. It's a gentle and easy way to regain a good night's rest.

PATIENTS FIND NIGHTLASE TO BE A HIGHLY COMFORTABLE AND SATISFYING SOLUTION.

Another measure of NightLase for the treatment of snoring would be your bed partner saying you're not snoring anymore. That's what we want. When I identify a patient as potentially having sleep apnea concerns, or sleep concerns, and they have been tested and evaluated by a sleep doctor and they're having snoring issues, NightLase can work miracles. And provide other miracles for improved partner relationships at night.

I queried a patient today about sleep, and he said, when my wife comes in, ask her how her snoring is. "Because it's pretty fierce," he said.

CPAP versus Oral Appliance Patient Compliance

We use the term *patient compliance* a little too much, in my opinion. It sounds like we have a demerit system or something. What compliance means, in dental speak, is the willingness and motivation of a patient to continue with treatment or therapy. So, that willingness to continue with oral appliances scores slightly higher than for CPAP and has been found to be between 60 and 70 percent after three years

of use. Not everybody loves them, but everybody loves to breathe well and sleep well.

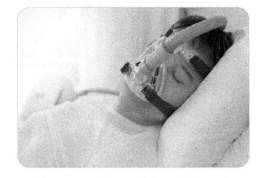

Patients used to have a surgical choice of a uvulectomy. The uvula (the small "punching bag" at the tip of the soft palate) often becomes enlarged if you have sleep apnea or snore. While the uvula rarely causes sleep apnea or snoring, it can contribute to both disorders. A head and neck surgeon may suggest removing a portion of the uvula known as a partial uvulectomy. Because complete uvulectomy has been associated with swallowing problems, drying of the throat, and the feeling of a lump in the throat, most surgeons no longer advocate the complete removal of the entire uvula. But even a partial procedure can be a difficult procedure.

Adults and Labial Frenectomy

We reviewed the frenectomy as regards children, but I must note that two out of every three labial frenectomies (tongue-ties) I perform are for adults. My well-rehearsed quiz in the dental chair asks: *How do you chew and swallow your food? How is your speech?* And of course, I will recognize that their speech is adaptive. Swallowing is important, because your tongue doesn't reach to the roof of your mouth far back to help aid with swallowing.

We see patients with narrowed arches. Even post-orthodontics, they can relapse, and then we'll ask: *Can you clear all of the molar spaces between your teeth and your cheeks and clear the food debris out of those spaces? Can you touch every tooth in your mouth, all surfaces with your tongue? The tip of your tongue?* And if you cannot do that, and you are restricted, then your body is not working to its maximum capacity. And there will be some downstream challenges.

During our procedure, we cut the fascia, a thin casing of connective tissue found throughout the body that surrounds and holds every organ, blood vessel, bone, nerve fiber, and muscle in place. It kind of holds everything up. If it's stressed, if it's tight, then your body's tight, like a guitar string. By releasing it, we can release some internal strains in the body. Recently, my patient subtly jumped in the chair when I cut the fascia, and she reported a feeling of tremendous release farther down in her body.

Years ago, we used to think that fascia tissue just covered organs, muscles, and bones. Now though, the medical world knows that the body's fascia also makes up some tendons, ligaments, and other structures, and some researchers believe that it connects all parts of the body.[96]

I think the advantageous frenectomy procedure is undervalued for adults. Many folks are skeptical about having this surgery for something that they've been adapted to for many, many years. We also

---

96   "Fascia: Layers, Pain, and Treatment," WebMD.com (WebMD, June 20, 2021), https://www.webmd.com/a-to-z-guides/what-is-fascia.

find some resistance to a sleep test. Many folks are a little intimidated by the notion of being wired up for a launch to Mars and then trying to go to sleep. Whatever the cause of the sleep disorder, some people comment that they've survived this long, doing it this way, so *why do I have to get a sleep test?*

Some are afraid that they're going to be diagnosed with some form of obstructive sleep apnea or sleep breathing disorders, and they may hear the word CPAP. If you hate that idea, you may oppose the sleep test. I did my sleep test when I was fifty-nine. I made sure my nose was okay. I try to do everything I can to prevent having to use a CPAP machine.

We can learn from the findings of the team at Walter Reed Army Institute of Research. They know the vital importance of sleep to maintain a squared-away emotional response to battle stress.

Sleeping helps regulate our emotional labeling. For soldiers who experience something traumatic, sleep will help them process events and reduce the chances of serious long-term emotional dysregulation, such as post-traumatic stress disorder (PTSD).

"If you were to be sleep deprived and experience something very emotional, the emotionality of it stays really high," the Walter Reed experts noted.

"But if you sleep, you save the memory, and the emotionality is slightly reduced."

The frontal lobe regulates emotions and processes events, and it does not function as effectively during periods of sleep deprivation. This means during stressful events, sleep-deprived individuals may perceive something as overly negative and respond disproportionally to the event.

"Our ability to translate what is a threat and not a threat and respond appropriately is critical, especially when you are working with the same team all the time, making decisions and regulating the perception of a threat," said Lt. Col. Vincent Capaldi, CMPN senior medical scientist.[97]

Colonel Capaldi added that there are experiences that will remain traumatic memories, however. "Taking the extra time to sleep and recover over several nights following a traumatic event will help to file your memories away in the proper place with the proper amount of emotional response from your brain, minimizing some effects of acute stress disorder and PTSD."

"Sleep debt doesn't necessarily create the pathologic conditions, but it can certainly make the pathological conditions worse, but if we get enough quality and quantity of sleep then we will mitigate a lot of the symptoms that are associated with these conditions," said Lt. Col. Scott Williams, CMPN director.[98]

Now transfer that wisdom to a typical American civilian career, stressed by the constant demand of showing up at work every day on time, unappreciative bosses, office politics, financial strain, unexpected job loss, the possible emotional toil of stressed relationships, difficult parenting, or toxic relationships.

Now keep going. Day after day. Get up tomorrow morning and get back on the horse. And we all hope you got some good sleep.

Just like the team that has been assembled to combat PTSD in the uniformed services, we too have set up such a team of diverse expertise to tackle sleep disorders. Dentists working collaboratively with primary care physicians and sleep specialists, as part of a multidisciplinary care team, can assist you in serving as the front line of

---

97   Gabriela Okhuysen, "Optimizing Sleep as a Soldier: The Science, Challenges and Significance," DVIDS (Walter Reed Army Institute of Research, October 28, 2021), https://www.dvidshub.net/news/408197/optimizing-sleep-soldier-science-challenges-and-significance.

98   Ibid.

defense for these difficult diagnostic dilemmas. We just need to be sure we get some regular nightly rest so we can be at our best.

The next chapter will help shape our understanding of how the sleep routine helps to detoxify our brain, and what we can do to help unblock our lymphatic system, freeing up the ability to recover from all the chin music (a pitched ball that passes very close to the batter's chin) that life can throw at us. I will extend that line of thought to the total body impact of clenching and our brain's need to detoxify nightly and how a jammed lymphatic system prevents this.

Without good sleep, nothing else works right. Dr. Maiken Nedergaard, a professor of neurosurgery at the University of Rochester explained this simply: "It's like a dishwasher." During sleep, a cleaning process is carried out where spinal fluid is pumped into the brain and removed at a rapid pace.

Upon waking the brain cells return to their enlarged state and the cerebrospinal fluid entering the brain turns to a trickle. Nedergaard says "It's almost like opening and closing a faucet." Until the glymphatic system was recognized and coined by Maiken Nedergaard, the absence of the lymphatic drainage pathway in the brain was puzzling.[99]

We refer to this as brain detoxification. *Because there's the rub.*

---

99   Biotics Research, "Detoxing the Brain: Sleep and Glymphatics," https://blog.bioticsresearch.com/detoxing-the-brain-sleep-and-glymphatics, accessed November 6, 2022.

DOES OUR BRAIN NEED TO BE DETOXED? LATHER, RINSE, REPEAT

Does our brain need to be detoxed? What's going on with our brain that would require it? This mostly happens during our deep restful sleep periods, but it happens a little bit during the day as well. We can support this through choices that we make, and we need to sometimes rev it up or de-sludge the toxins in our brain with some dental intervention. And whoa, what does a dentist have that can help with that?

And really, what would be some of the symptoms of these toxins? We can recall our review of the symptoms of brain fog or lack of clarity and thought and just not thinking properly. Well, I do know that if we don't take the garbage out all the time, it's going to build up, and then it's going to smell and generally create an unpleasant environment. If our brain doesn't detoxify properly, we get this buildup going on in there.

*"It's probably equally important that when you are awake, you
be really awake. If you are bored all day, that is not good for you
either. You need to enjoy life and then switch off for the night."*

Those wise words are from one of the world's top scientists, Maiken Nedergaard MD, DMSc, best known as the discoverer of the brain's sleep-time cleansing mechanism—a game changer in our understanding of why we need to sleep and a key step in the understanding of how brain diseases such as Alzheimer's begin.

DR. MAIKEN NEDERGAARD IS AMONG THE WORLD'S TOP 1 PERCENT OF CITED RESEARCHERS.

Dr. Maiken Nedergaard is among the world's top 1 percent of cited researchers.

In 2013, when this brilliant Danish neuroscientist discovered the glymphatic system, we awakened to the realization that a network of channels in the brain eliminates toxins using cerebrospinal fluid (CSF). She called it the "glymphatic system" due to its dependence on glial cells, which enable our brain to clear itself nightly if we get good sleep. She swept back the bedcovers to reveal a formerly unknown layer of understanding about all life forms: why we all need to sleep.

She serves as professor of neurosurgery, neuroscience and neurology, and co-director of the Center for Translational Neuromedicine at the University of Copenhagen, in Denmark, where she is a professor of glial cell biology. Dr. Nedergaard also serves as a jointly appointed professor in the departments of neuroscience and neurology at the University of Rochester Medical Center.

Toxic

I pause to apologize for the use of a word that has been so stretched in meaning that we hardly know how to describe it, the word *toxic*.

Because of the widespread use for almost anything negative, *toxic* won the gold star and became the stand-out choice for the 2018 Oxford Word of the Year title. We hear about toxic work environments, toxic relationships, toxic metals, toxic politics, and toxic environments. Well, it seems less frightening than the word *poisonous.*

Because of the groundbreaking work of Dr. Maiken Nedergaard, we know that during sleep, our brain volume decreases, and it creates channels or spaces that fill up with cerebral spinal fluid. Then through a gradient difference, the cells dump their proteins, toxins, and cellular byproducts across the membrane, into the lymph system, which transports it downstream until we excrete it. Scientists studying the onset of dementia refer to the "amyloid buildup" in our brain, which can be a marker for Alzheimer's.

We can visualize the "osmosis" that occurs, the name for the flow of fluids when there's a difference in concentrations, through a semi-permeable membrane. Fluids flow from an area of high concentration to an area of low concentration. Our brain pumps out the cells that have a high concentration of toxins, passing them through the membrane. If that cellular membrane becomes damaged, perhaps by inflammation in our body, this easy passageway in and out of the cells can be affected.

In fact, Dr. Laura Lewis, a professor of biomedical engineering at Boston University, said in a statement that in 2019, she and her colleagues had captured images of sleeping brains by having thirteen research participants, all in their twenties and thirties, fall asleep in a magnetic resonance imaging (MRI) machine.[100]

"The participants, who were paid for this uncomfortable arrangement, also had to wear a net of electrodes on their scalps to measure

---

100   Stephanie Pappas, "Watch Spinal Fluid 'Wash' the Sleeping Brain in Rhythmic, Pulsing Waves," Live Science, accessed October 17, 2022, https://www.livescience.com/cerebrospinal-fluid-washes-sleeping-brain.html.

the electrical activity of their brains. The results showed a pulsing, predictable flow. First, neural activity quiets. Then, blood flows out of the brain. Next, cerebrospinal fluid flows in. Lather, rinse, repeat. The pattern is so consistent that it's possible to just look at cerebrospinal fluid in a given brain region and tell whether a person is awake or asleep," Lewis said.

Researchers from the Nedergaard group at the University of Rochester Medical Center spent years uncovering how healthy lifestyle choices translate into better brain function. In a study published in January 2018 in *Neuroscience Letters*, Dr. Nedergaard's team demonstrated that exercise helps clear away harmful debris in the brain.

"A VERY EXPENSIVE ORGAN"

In a recent blog titled "Clearing Out the Junk: Healthy Lifestyle Choices Boost Brain Waste Disposal," by the Harvard Graduate School of Arts and Sciences writer Benjamin Andreone, he depicted the brain as "a very expensive organ."

"Although it takes up only 2 percent of the body's mass, it uses about 20 percent of its total energy to work efficiently. While this high energy demand allows us to sense our world, communicate with one another, and remember how to get to work each morning, it, unfortunately, comes at a cost," Andreone said.

Andreone explained all this very clearly.

He added that "when brain cells called neurons consume high amounts of energy, they spit out a lot of debris that floats around the brain and prevents it from functioning normally. This debris consists mostly of leftover proteins, which when left alone, can form clumps that are toxic to the brain."[101]

---

101   Benjamin Andreone, "Clearing Out the Junk: Healthy Lifestyle Choices Boost Brain Waste Disposal," Harvard University Graduate School of Arts and Sciences, accessed October 14, 2022, https://sitn. hms.harvard.edu/flash/2018/clearing-junk-healthy-lifestyle-choices-boost-brain-waste-disposal/.

In particular, he noted, clumping of the protein *amyloid beta* has been linked to decreases in cognition, memory, and overall brain function in people with Alzheimer's. In most organs of the body, the lymphatic system acts as a waste disposal factory to clear away harmful debris.

"The lymphatic system—comprised primarily of an extensive series of vessels that traverse the body—produces a fluid called lymph. Lymph flows through each organ, mops up debris, and washes it into a network of ducts that eventually drain into blood vessels. Once in the blood, the debris travels on to the kidneys and liver, where it is eliminated from the body,"[102] Andreone concludes.

Decreasing the toxic load in our body reduces the inflammation that can be directly related to nighttime grinding or bruxing. When we lose more than three millimeters of tooth height from grinding, it will decrease our ability to properly detox in the glial system by about 50 percent. The more clenching, the more grinding, the more your teeth wear, the less your brain detoxes. That affects sleep a lot.

We should note the effect of pain on sleep. If clenching, you can develop cervical and facial pain because the muscles are being abused or used too heavily. And in pain, your body cannot sleep well because of the arousal at night by this.

When new technologies like the Oura ring measure sleep quality, the number of arousals certainly becomes part of the calculation determining how well your body can get into a deep sleep. You're not sleeping well if you are constantly being poked by clenching and facial pain. It's a vicious cycle. Compensate by having less pain in the TMJ or the muscle surrounding it by trying a night guard to see if that causes some decompression in that area.

---

102   Ibid.

"You ... Have Fire."

I remember well the day of my son Brian's examination and treatment for his Lyme disease by a very devoted acupuncturist, a Chinese practitioner with broken English.

She looked at Brian's beet-red tongue. And she looked at him, and then me, and said in almost unintelligible broken English, "You have ... fire."

An enlightening moment for my ideological evolution, it had taken me a long time to understand that something burning inside him struggled to come out, and we had to squash that fire through multiple modalities, like acupuncture, diet modification, meditation, breath work, exercise, and supplements. Most importantly, now I knew that to quench this fire, we would need all of these and more.

Years later, I had my own encounter with COVID-19. For several days, my brain seemed a little bit off. The elevator did not quite make it to the top floor. My crispness and my thought process definitely suffered. I needed to do something. I needed to put out the fire. I needed to detox or let's say *get the lymph moving*, try to get a better night's sleep, try to clear my head, make sure that I did not clench, and remain alert to breathe properly. I benefited from the earlier VivAer procedure, and my nasal passages stayed super clear.

I clearly recall my ENT physician inserting a small VivAer wand into my nostrils to precisely target and treat the blockage. The tip of the wand uses low-temperature radiofrequency (RF) energy to gently remodel your nasal passage to improve airflow.

I could breathe freely through my nose. I did not walk around with my mouth wide open, a good thing for me. Clear breathing, while awake or asleep, wins half the battle.

Healthy Lifestyle

Whether fighting off a virus, or just trying to reduce brain fog, we want these byproducts removed. We do not want to develop these neurological or neurocognitive issues. We need enough good sleep. Diet remains really important, a less toxic, organic-based diet where we put fewer bad things into our body. To use a metaphor we can all understand, we should put "good hi-test gas" into our vehicles. Healthy fats are important. Our night should be in a dark room environment, free of noise, allowing our body to produce melatonin. An increase in exercise increases glial activity. An increase in hydration helps support the gradient differentials and keep the interstitial fluids filled. Increase your cognitive muscle by staying mentally active.

As the world becomes more toxic (*there's that word again, sorry*), we have an increase in brain illnesses like Parkinson's and Alzheimer's. COVID-19, on the other hand, presents a systemic inflammatory body reaction. Your cells become inflamed, in fact, your organs can become inflamed.

Inflammation is like a fire in your body you cannot see or feel. Harvard Medical School weighs in:

"It's a smoldering process that injures your tissues, joints, and blood vessels, and you often do not notice it until significant damage is done," says Dr. Andrew Luster, of the Center for Immunology and Inflammatory Diseases at Harvard-affiliated Massachusetts General Hospital. The damage might show up as arthritis, heart disease, stroke, and even Alzheimer's disease."[103]

That's one reason people are on ventilators. Their lungs are fighting off inflammation in the body, trying to *put out the fires.*

---

103 "Playing with the Fire of Inflammation," https://www.health.harvard.edu/ (Harvard Health Publishing, April 12, 2021), https://www.health.harvard.edu/staying-healthy/playing-with-the-fire-of-inflammation.

Melatonin and Immunity

Dr. Maiken Nedergaard confirmed that the brain plays a vital role in our immune system. As we sleep, our brain cells decrease by 60 percent, which supports drainage. Melatonin, one of the most important molecules for clearing the brain, represents our main antioxidant up there and detox agent for mercury, lead, aluminum, and other heavy metals. Melatonin helps stimulate our lymphatic system. We need to have proper melatonin production. Good sleep hygiene becomes vital in all this.

When we chew, the muscles in our face pump our lymphatics. We found through research that if we experience an increase in toxins, there's a decrease in melatonin, which affects our sleep, a vicious circle.

Harvard writer Benjamin Andreone asked Dr. Nedergaard if she takes sleep more seriously since her discovery, something she probably got precious little of while her five children were young, despite her claiming they were all good sleepers. "Oh yes, I have a whole sleep routine," she chuckled. "It drives my husband crazy."[104]

It's all in a good night's sleep.

---

104   Benjamin Andreone, "Clearing Out the Junk: Healthy Lifestyle Choices Boost Brain Waste Disposal," Harvard University Graduate School of Arts and Sciences, accessed October 14, 2022, https://sitn. hms.harvard.edu/flash/2018/clearing-junk-healthy-lifestyle-choices-boost-brain-waste-disposal/.

TRY THESE TIPS FOR A BETTER, MORE REFRESHING REST[105]

MAINTAIN A REGULAR BEDTIME

Going to bed (and waking up) at approximately the same time every day can help you get better rest and improve your overall sleep quality.

CONSIDER YOUR DIET

Eating certain foods, especially later in the day, may disrupt your sleep. For better sleep, try to avoid the following just before bedtime:

- large meals
- heavy or rich foods
- spicy and acidic foods
- caffeine (including chocolate)
- alcohol

If you feel hungry before bedtime, try a better bedtime snack, such as:

- a banana
- yogurt
- a small bowl of oatmeal
- cheese, fruit, and crackers

CREATE A COMFORTABLE SLEEPING ENVIRONMENT

Keeping your bedroom cool and dark can help you get better sleep. If you tend to get warm or cold during the night, opt for layers of light-weight, breathable bedding.

SET ASIDE SOME DE-STRESS TIME BEFORE BED

Stress and anxiety are both common culprits behind sleep issues. Being available to relax before bed won't necessarily get rid of these concerns, but it can help you put them out of your mind for the evening.

---

105 Crystal Raypole, "How to 'Detox' Your Brain (Hint: It's Easier Than You Think)," Healthline, accessed October 14, 2020, https://www.healthline.com/health/brain-detox#takeaway.

An hour or so before bedtime, try:

- Journaling about stressors.

- Writing out things you need to take care of the next day, so you won't worry about them.

- Coloring, reading, or other calming activities.

- Taking a warm bath with candles or aromatherapy.

- Doing some light yoga or meditating.

- Deep breathing exercises.

EXERCISE PLAYS A BIG ROLE TOO

You know that refreshed, focused feeling (despite your tired muscles) after a big workout? That's the glymphatic system kicking in.

TAKE TIME TO RELAX

Mental breaks are just as important as physical breaks. Make sure you're regularly giving your brain a rest by setting aside some time to simply sit and enjoy the moment. This will allow your brain to recharge and boost your creative energy. Your brain will thank you.

Source: *Healthline*, "How to 'Detox' Your Brain (Hint: It's Easier Than You Think)"

Lymphatic Remedy

We have found significant success using a series of injections of a preservative-free non-epinephrine anesthetic down the lymphatic chain, in and around the TMJ, behind the ears and in front of the ears, and down the neck. This popular neural therapy technique stimulates the lymph in that area to re-engage it and makes it less stagnant.

Recently, I worked with a team of New York City physicians on neural therapy for several of their patients. We performed injections to relax the autonomic nervous system to influence the parasympathetic nervous system. Our goal was to relieve pain in certain parts of the body through the use of these injections, mostly in the head and neck. Later, I used the same technique we developed in New York on a patient suffering from TMD and a foggy feeling in her head. We did cervical lymphatics chain injections followed by ozone, and it helped the lymphatic systems to drain better, while providing a calming, relaxing feeling for the patient.

Focusing on the TMJ, neck, and under the mandible, we work to reduce muscle activity around the jaw until it's not clenching as much. Using this series of injections creates a clearing of this brain fog. Many issues with Lyme and even migraines can be dealt with using these neurotherapy techniques.

Pain

People tend to brux when they are in pain, and folks tend to brux about 50 percent of the time when they're not breathing properly. We must fix the nose if it limits the proper oxygen. My academic colleagues often characterize bruxism as a sleep disorder, but I would suggest that it demonstrates a *sleep movement* disorder, a central nervous system issue, and has a lot to do, I believe, with not breathing properly at night and not getting enough oxygen. I refer hundreds of patients for sleep studies because often, the bottom line reveals the inability to breathe properly through the nose at night. Once a patient has their sleep test and they do not have moderate or severe apnea, we can consider laser NightLase procedures and a sleep appliance.

There are fewer traditional tools for unclogging the lymphatic system, which I have mentioned earlier, such as Dr. Tennant's Bio-Modulator. I have a dental unit in my office that I use to treat stiffness in the jaw muscles, for TMJ, and post-extraction therapies. Treatments last about twenty minutes. They either hold it, or it's on a microphone stand. But if the patient has systemic issues, I refer them to the Tennant Institute.

We refer patients to Dr. Tennant for the use of this technology to ensure normal and healthy voltage, assuring that the cells have the proper voltage to do their jobs efficiently. Then, pads and plates are applied to your head and neck to help with healing, pain, and stiffness of the TMJ and surrounding muscles.

I often recommend low-laser light therapy (LLLT) for photo biomodulation to stimulate and improve the mitochondria inside the cells, enabling the cells to have the proper energy to work. Pulse electromagnetic field (PEMF) therapy is an adjunct therapy, which can reduce inflammation, reduce pain, and help bring the body back to a normal state.

Pineal Gland and Melatonin

If you take oral melatonin, know that it pales in comparison to the natural melatonin your body produces in the pineal gland, a small, pea-sized, pinecone-shaped endocrine structure near the center of the brain. We know the importance of melatonin for sleep. Now we know pineal melatonin can protect against neurodegeneration, the progressive loss of function of neurons, present in conditions such as Alzheimer's disease and Parkinson's disease.

But because the pineal gland resides outside of the blood-brain barrier, it's more vulnerable and susceptible to damage from environmental toxins, heavy metals, and other pollutants. Aluminum, fluoride, glyphosate, and mercury can all cause damage to this gland and decrease our melatonin production. The choices of materials and treatments that dentists use for patients take on a more intense urgency.

The Cleveland Clinic reports that researchers have found that people who've had their pineal gland surgically removed (pinealectomy) experienced an accelerated aging process. Because of this, some scientists think natural melatonin may have anti-aging properties.[106]

Cranial Sacral Work

Cranial sacral therapy (CST), sometimes referred to as craniosacral therapy, refers to a type of bodywork that relieves compression in the bones of the head, sacrum (a triangular bone in the lower back), and spinal column.

A physical therapist and other health professionals can perform CST. The therapist uses gentle pressure on the head, neck, and back to relieve the discomfort caused by compression. As a result, it can help treat several conditions with gentle manipulation and offers another modality to help move, get the brain pulsing properly, and get the lymphatic drainage happening.

If not breathing properly through your nose, you can unconsciously have your nose up in the air, your head canted forward a little bit. This puts strain on the cervical part of your neck. Or if you're a computer tech person looking down a lot, this puts pressure on that system, too. It's being compressed in certain areas. Head posture can be evaluated through X-ray evaluation by chiropractors and physicians. Sometimes the 3D CT scan reveals these issues. Neck pain and headaches are the usual symptoms.

---

106   "Melatonin: What It Is & Function," https://my.clevelandclinic.org/ (Cleveland Clinic, July 5, 2022), https://my.clevelandclinic.org/health/articles/23411-melatonin.

Herbals

While I am not an herbalist, I suggest some herbal remedies for clenching problems.

My son used melatonin with his Lyme disease because his sleeping became poor. He couldn't sleep because his sympathetic nervous system kicked into overdrive. Our sympathetic nervous system responds to dangerous or stressful situations. In these situations, the sympathetic nervous system activates to speed up your heart rate and deliver more blood to areas of your body that need more oxygen or other responses to help us escape danger.

His body wasn't being given a chance to relax. Cleveland Clinic notes that your sympathetic nervous system "takes the lead when your safety and survival are at risk, but that system's actions can strain body systems when it's active for too long. Because these two systems offset each other, they help maintain balance in your body."[107]

Getting your body back into a parasympathetic process makes all the sense in the world, and magnesium is a great supplement. The most popular bathing salts are Epsom salts and magnesium flakes, which contain magnesium compounds in different forms. Magnesium benefits are world renowned for aiding sleep quality and relieving muscle tension.

Take a twenty-minute, toasty-warm bath one night and see what I mean. While you're soaking in your bath salts, peruse the next chapter on how healthy behaviors such as this can help prevent having some severe problems with your gut health. (When we use the word *gut*, we refer to the entire intestinal tract.)

---

107   "Parasympathetic Nervous System (PSNS)," my.clevelandclinic.com (Cleveland Clinic, June 6, 2022), https://my.clevelandclinic.org/health/body/23266-parasympathetic-nervous-system-psns.

PERIODONTAL DISEASE AND GUT HEALTH

A High-Speed, Nonstop Train That Runs Both Ways

If you remain unconvinced that the condition of your teeth and gums can make a significant impact on your overall health, this chapter should convince you that your skepticism is misplaced.

Periodontal disease, commonly known as gum disease, can cause bleeding gums and bad breath, and if left untreated, lead to tooth loss. Research from the AAP and the Centers for Disease Control and Prevention suggests that up to half of US adults aged thirty and older have some form of periodontal disease. Periodontal disease has been linked to several other severe conditions, including diabetes, heart disease, and Alzheimer's.

U.S. News & World Report reported in 2022 that researchers in Finland, in a review of forty-seven previously published studies, found that tooth loss, deep pockets around teeth in the gums, or bone loss in the tooth sockets was tied to a 21 percent higher risk of dementia and a 23 percent higher risk of milder cognitive decline.[108]

New research published in the *Journal of Clinical Periodontology* links periodontitis and COVID-19 complications.[109] The American Academy of Periodontology (AAP) warned in the winter of 2021 that systemic inflammation may indicate COVID-19 "but can also be a symptom of periodontal disease or gum disease."

Farther down the intestinal tract, we can have a leaky gut issue or gut dysbiosis for many reasons, led by the toxins in the typical American diet, which break down the lining of the intestinal tract. And when that happens, it leaks the bacteria into your blood system, and your blood system has to figure out what to do with that. We want to maintain the lining of our stomach and intestines because that's how we clear our bodies of waste and toxins.

And if we break the integrity of the intestinal lining, we can cause a systemic, chronic issue of body inflammation. If we have systemic inflammation, that can show itself in our gum tissues and mouth. That becomes an issue because the junction around each tooth opens to toxins, foods, sugar, and bad fats. And that leaks into our system, into our blood. And it causes havoc.

Not only havoc, but it also causes us to have local infections in the jawbone, maybe into the nerves of the teeth. We could call this periodontal disease a leaky mouth. Leaky gut. Leaky mouth. Devoted clinical researchers keep finding evidence that we probably have periodontal disease if we have a leaky gut.

---

108   Steven Reinberg, "Unhealthy Gums Could up Your Odds for Dementia," usnews.com (US News & World Report, September 12, 2022), https://www.usnews.com/news/health-news/articles/2022-09-12/unhealthy-gums-could-up-your-odds-for-dementia.

109   "New Study Links Periodontitis and Covid-19 Complications," perio.org (American Academy of Periodontology, February 3, 2021), https://www.perio.org/press-release/new-study-links-periodontitis-and-covid%E2%80%9019-complications/.

A systemic reaction can show up in the mouth. It's a two-way railroad. If the digestive lining breaks down, we can see signs of periodontal disease in the mouth. It goes both ways on a high-speed track. Gum disease can mirror the inflammatory condition of the body as a whole. It takes part in a two-way or bi-directional relationship. Inflammation of the mouth mirrors and contributes to the inflammation of the body. Conversely, the inflammation of the body mirrors and contributes to the inflammation of the mouth.

Dental Treatment of Periodontal Disease

Biomedical Journal reports that periodontal disease or gum disease has become the most prevalent disease in the mouth. Quite simply, gum disease results from inflammation of the gums around your teeth that goes unchecked or is not treated correctly.[110]

When dentists treat their patients, we also often treat the related structures. We can comfortably stay within our scope of work to get into the problems caused by diet. How do we treat all that? We follow a couple of different paths. We do localized therapies, such as deep scaling. It depends on the condition. Patients can have gingivitis, all the way down to bone loss, periodontal disease, or periodontitis. The amount of lost tissue will give us an indication of how long this systemic inflammatory problem has been going on.

And a better diet, a purer diet, can help everything, a hard thing to do in today's society because of the ease of opening up the fridge and grabbing some processed foods. Higher food prices limit many folks from buying organic products.

---

110   Fiona Q. Bui, Cassio Almeida-da-Silva, Brandon Huynh, Alston Trinh, "Association between Periodontal Pathogens and Systemic Disease," *Biomedical Journal* (March 2019).

A poor diet can cause pathogenic microbes in our stomach to overgrow and cause damage.

"I like to think of the microbiome as a three-to-five-pound garden that we have living inside of us," Dr. Elroy Vojdani of Regenera Medical in Los Angeles, told Healthline.

"What you feed that garden dictates what type of plants grow in that garden. If you feed it fuel that supports anti-inflammatory healthy bacteria, such as plant-based fibers and plant-based fats then you get a garden that has healthy, good bacteria and yeast living inside of it," he explained. "If you feed the garden processed foods, sugar, and animal fat, then weeds will grow in that garden. Essentially, it's a living and breathing biomass that is very responsive to what you put into it. When you put in healthy things, you get healthy things out."[111]

Generally speaking, fast foods are the unhealthiest for the gut. Plant-based foods are recommended. Stay away from burgers and fries as much as is humanly possible.

Bleeding Gums and Why We Have Cavities

Bleeding gums act like the proverbial canary in the coal mine. We have a jumpstart on this process because of the work of Dr. R. R. Steinman and Dr. John Lenora, who published a breakthrough study in late 1971 to help us figure out why we have cavities. They suggested that there exists a dental fluid transport system.

They studied the disease from the pulpal (dentinal fluid) side instead of only attributing it to the acid destruction of the tooth by a hostile microenvironment. Dr. Steinman and Dr. Lenora recognized the importance of a dynamic fluid transport mechanism and linked

---

111   Christopher Curley, "Fast Foods Harm Your Gut Microbiome: What You Should Eat Instead," Healthline, April 22, 2021, https://www.healthline.com/health-news/fast-foods-harm-your-gut-microbiome-what-you-should-eat-instead.

its functionality to physiological mechanisms. They wanted to figure out why we have cavities. Parents want to know why their kids have all these cavities, even kids that may not take in much sugar.[112]

They performed animal studies to see if sugar directly causes cavities. But interestingly, they found that a tooth is porous. The pulp chamber, in the middle of the tooth, has a blood supply. Then it moves out into the dentinal tubules and goes into the tooth's enamel. When healthy, our teeth have nourishing fluids flowing from the dental pulp outward through the tubules, enamel, and mouth. The tooth's juices flow out. That keeps the cavities away, and the scientists named this process *dentinal fluid transport*.[113]

These fluids continuously flow out from the dental pulp outward through the dentinal tubules and enamel and into the mouth protecting our teeth. They inhibit acids, prevent harmful organisms from getting inside the tooth, and provide a proper pH balance to neutralize bacterial acids. The researchers noted that it's only when this transport system experiences a malfunction that cavities form. Decay can begin when the fluid flow is interrupted. Bacteria attack the tooth when resistance weakens.

Dr. Clyde Roggenkamp, DDS, MSD, MPH, was a student of Ralph Steinman, DDS, and John Leonora, PhD, at Loma Linda University School of Dentistry. In 2005, Dr. Roggenkamp published a brilliant book about the life work of his mentors.

Their findings had met ho-hum resistance from the dental community at the time, not unlike the mercury amalgam issue. (Though, the work by these scientists was ignored for only a few years, not decades like the amalgam wars.)

---

112   R. R. Steinman, J. Leonora, "Relationship of Fluid Transport through the Dentin to the Incidence of Dental Caries," *Journal of Dental Research* (November-December 1971), https://pubmed.ncbi.nlm.nih.gov/5288889.

113   Ibid.

An alert graduate student, Clyde Roggenkamp, DDS, MSD, MPH, dove into the shelved studies, authoring his own book about it.

"With perseverance and bit by bit, they designed beautiful experiments in an attempt to tear down that wall," he said, and because of his efforts, this theory has found new traction in our work.

In the book *Dentinal Fluid Transport*, Dr. Roggenkamp and co-writer John Lenora, MD, revived intelligent discussion about the innate hormone-regulated fluid transport mechanism that has been shown ordinarily to fend off decay-producing acid and aid enamel and dentinal caries resistance. This research repeatedly demonstrated control of this natural caries-preventive mechanism to become disrupted by high dietary sugar at the systemic level. This interference may provide the ultimate cause of dental caries.[114]

Sugar?

Sugar causes cavities. But wait, there's more …

Everybody's taught us that we must brush our teeth, floss our teeth (only floss the ones you want to keep), and stay away from sugar. We do all this, but we also need to stay away from carbohydrates because those fermentable carbohydrates turn into sugar, changing our mouth's pH, and becoming more acidic.

The acidic byproduct of the bacteria lays against the tooth, breaking down the enamel and causing decay. But we're finding that if our body has this flow from inside the tooth outward through proper pH and blood chemistry pH, we will have fewer cavities than if our body faces a more acidic environment where this fluid transport system reverses. It brings all the toxins and acidic byproducts from the

---

114   "Clyde L. Roggenkamp, DDS, MSD," https://llu.edu/ (Loma Linda University), accessed February 7, 2023, https://home.llu.edu/academics/faculty/roggenkamp-clyde/research.

bacteria and plaque into the tooth and breaks down the enamel, causing cavities.

That has a lot to do with how we eat. If we eat well, our gastrointestinal tract does not become inflamed, and we don't have a leaky gut. We will not develop periodontal disease or leaky mouth and will have less systemic inflammation.

I still marvel at this miraculous dental fluid transport system. When we introduce sugar into the mouth, the parotid gland excretes sodium bicarbonate and tries to neutralize the acidity inside the mouth. These scientists figured that it's not necessarily the bacteria and the sugar intake, but it's more systemic in regulating decay. What a fantastic system of balancing our body provides us.

High sugar intake reverses dental fluid transport. If you're sucking on carbonated sodas, candy bars all day, or carbs, it changes the flow toward the tooth. A lack of micronutrients can cause this reversal, and medicines can also do it. We still know that sugar has some guilt here; carbohydrates also sneak around. They have a lot to do with it. If we eat all that tasty stuff, we put our bodies in a more stressful situation.

We have found that if our body has a healthy flow from inside the tooth outward through a proper blood chemistry pH, we will have fewer cavities and see a close relationship to the body's pH.

Stress can also interrupt the dental fluid transport system. Emotional anxiety, physical stress, and long-term lack of exercise play a significant role because exercise burns up sugar, reducing the sugar in your mouth and body. Then it complicates other critical systems in the body. How do we attack it? We attack it in two ways: simultaneously

> **WE'RE FINDING THAT IF OUR BODY HAS THIS FLOW FROM INSIDE THE TOOTH OUTWARD, WE WILL HAVE FEWER CAVITIES THAN IF THIS FLUID TRANSPORT SYSTEM REVERSES.**

by cleaning out the infection in the mouth and motivating the patient to improve their diet.

> *"The human body contains almost as many*
> *bacterial cells as human cells."*[115]

We perform a deep scaling or debridement to clean out the infection in the gum tissues. We may find infection in the bone, or the gum tissues and localized hard plaque called tartar or calculus. We try to remove that as well. Laser technology has become one of the most efficient ways of doing it in today's world. I use my Fotona laser. That cleans out the infection and helps stimulate the mitochondria in the tissues to promote regrowth and a healthier environment. We get that laser energy deep into the tissues and some into the bone where the bacteria like to hide.

Fixing the Diet

We also suggest ways to fix the stomach or your gut. Dentists need to counsel their patients on a diet as much as possible. Move the toxins out of the body.

Visiting the dentist for periodontal therapy should include a close look at how we eat and how we can repopulate the healthy bacteria in our gut by feeding the beneficial bacteria with prebiotics and fiber.

All this directly relates to our gum health because we know that it causes periodontal disease. Anaerobic bacteria (porphyromonas gingivalis) is found in the mouth and through leaky gum tissue; they migrate via the blood stream to other parts of the body. They can be found in our brains. They cause cardiovascular issues. They could

---

115   R. Sender, S. Fuchs, R. Milo, "Are We Really Vastly Outnumbered? Revisiting the Ratio of Bacterial to Host Cells in Humans," *Cell*, January 13, 2016.

thrive in our stomachs because we're chronically swallowing them, and those harmful bacteria impact our health.

Most people think my dietary advice will be, *Don't eat as much sugar or overprocessed carbohydrates.* True. Those sugar and overprocessed carbohydrates can worsen your gut dysbiosis, creating a vicious cycle between your stomach, gums, and gum health.

We also want to try replacing an unhealthy processed diet with a nutritious anti-inflammatory diet. But how do we begin? I tell my patients to shop the *perimeter of the supermarket*, where we find vegetables, fruits, lean meats, and maybe even some cheeses. I advise against nutrient-deficient boxed foods made to taste better because they put in excess sugar and chemicals. I try to motivate my patients to eat a nutrient-dense, anti-inflammatory diet.

An inattentive dietary life results in a bit of sludge and slowdown caused by the mucus layer in our gut. We need to make sure that's healthy. Unfortunately, many dairy products stimulate mucus. And these products, especially if they're not hormone-free and pasteurized, may not represent what we want to feed our family. That causes mucus. That can become a very acidic pH problem, causing inflammation. Our body needs to be more pH neutral or alkaline to stay healthy. If it becomes chronically acidic, that corrodes the body's tissue, leading to systemic inflammation.

This subject brings out the environmentalist in me. With these dairy products, we take into our bodies exactly what the actual cow eats. That could include corn products, which can have glyco-phosphates, from GMO (genetically modified organism) corn. And that's what the cow's eating. We consume the cow as well as cow byproducts.

We will all likely eat foods and products made with ingredients from GMO crops. We liberally use these GMO crops to make ingredients Americans eat, such as cornstarch, corn syrup, soybean oil, canola oil, or granulated sugar. We can find fresh fruit and vegetables in GMO varieties, including potatoes, summer squash, apples, papayas, and pink pineapples. Although GMOs silently reside in many foods we eat, most of the GMO crops grown in the United States go into animal food.

Our governments have okayed all this while we sort out the impact of this relatively new genetic manipulation of our environment. As a passionate environmentalist, I do not like genetic engineering of any kind. This trend could end up being a disaster. Who will be held accountable for this when the nightmare scenarios arrive? *What were we thinking?*

We genetically engineer up to 92 percent of US corn, 94 percent of soybeans, and 94 percent of cotton. (Cottonseed oil is often used in food products.) It has been estimated that over 75 percent of processed foods on supermarket shelves—from soda to soup, crackers to condiments—contain genetically engineered ingredients.

The Center for Food Safety has been at the forefront of organizing a powerful food movement fighting the industrial model and promoting organic, ecological, and sustainable alternatives.

Their viewpoint raises red flags we have not seen coming.

> *By removing the genetic material from one organism and inserting it into the permanent genetic code of another, the biotech industry has created an astounding number of organisms that are not produced by nature and have never been seen on the plate. These include potatoes with bacteria genes, 'super' pigs with human growth genes, fish with cattle growth genes, tomatoes with flounder genes, corn with bacteria genes, and thousands of other altered and engineered plants, animals, and insects. At an alarming rate, these creations are now being patented and released into our environment and food supply.*[116]

116 "About Genetically Engineered Foods," https://www.centerforfoodsafety.org/ (Center for Food Safety), accessed February 7, 2023, https://www.centerforfoodsafety.org/issues/311/ge-foods/about-ge-foods.

BIOENGINEERED FOODS THAT OUR GOVERNMENTS HAVE AUTHORIZED FOR COMMERCIAL PRODUCTION

- Alfalfa, apple (ArcticTM varieties)

- Canola

- Corn

- Cotton

- Eggplant (BARI Bt Begun varieties)

- Papaya (ringspot virus-resistant varieties)

- Pineapple (pink-fleshed varieties)

- Potato

- Salmon (AquAdvantage)

- Soybean

- Summer squash

- Sugarbeet[117]

Overprocessed, high sugar, high carbohydrate diets cause the body to go into a more acidic environment, which causes inflammation in your stomach, which causes inflammation in your mouth, in other organs, things like brain fog or anxiety, allergies, food sensitivities, fatigue, joint and muscle pain, skin lesions, and pimples.

The body will rebel. *Hey, I'm not happy here.* Many folks think they'll *get over it,* and our bodies compensate. The body compensates for a while ... until it doesn't.

---

117   "GMO Crops, Animal Food, and Beyond," https://www.fda.gov/ (U.S. Food and Drug Administration, August 3, 2022), https://www.fda.gov/food/agricultural-biotechnology/gmo-crops-animal-food-and-beyond.

How do we balance our diet? Many diets advocate less acidic processed foods and more alkaline foods, and your body will respond well to that.

On August 31, 2022, Alison Aubrey of NPR published a frank and enlightening story headlined, "U.S. Diet Is Deadly. Here Are Seven Ideas to Get Americans Eating Healthier."

"The data are stark," she reports. "The typical American diet is shortening the lives of many Americans. Diet-related deaths outrank deaths from smoking, and about half of US deaths from heart disease—nearly 900 deaths a day—are linked to poor diet. The pandemic highlighted the problem, with much worse outcomes for people with obesity and other diet-related diseases."[118]

Alison Aubrey's story suggests that the US is in "a nutrition crisis in this country."

One of the innovative societal changes she recommends is to "focus on the quality of calories, not just quantity."

"The U.S. food supply is awash in cheap calories. And when you're on a tight budget or relying on benefits like SNAP (food stamps), processed foods like chips and soda can set you back less than fresh produce."

"Of course, eating processed foods also contributes to cardio-vascular disease, stroke, diabetes, and other chronic illnesses, warns Nancy Brown, CEO of the American Heart Association. Brown said federal food assistance programs have helped to address hunger. "However, many US food policies and programs focus on improving access to sufficient quantities of food," she says. Instead, it's time to

---

118   Alison Aubrey, "The U.S. Diet Is Deadly. Here Are 7 Ideas to Get Americans Eating Healthier," NPR, August 31, 2022, https://www.npr.org/sections/health-shots/2022/08/31/1120004717/the-u-s-diet-is-deadly-here-are-7-ideas-to-get-americans-eating-healthier.

modernize these policies and focus on food quality "so people have access to enough nutritious food."[119]

I usually suggest that my patients visit a nutritionist or naturopath for the best diet.

Proper pH contributes significantly to our bone health. From the dentist's point of view, we need excellent bone health to place implants. Your physician can take the pH of your blood. Your blood has a normal pH range of 7.35 to 7.45. This means that healthy blood chemistry tests report as slightly alkaline or basic. The closer your pH gets to 7.365, the higher your level of health.

We can use oral DNA testing to know precisely what mouth bacteria are present. This information enables us to predict a patient's susceptibility to certain periodontal diseases and tooth decay. It also allows us to treat the mouth before certain bacteria cause severe and permanent damage.

We must ensure that your body has the proper balance for long-term success or initial success of placing implants, doing traditional periodontal bone surgery, or trying to promote some reattachment using the laser. We have succeeded in regrowing some of the bone around a tooth using the laser's energy, killing the bacteria, changing the environment, and trying to put somebody on a good diet.

A yeast infection called *Candida* appears in the mouth due to an improper diet. It shows on the tongue or in the throat, or in the mucosa of the mouth. We can test the pH through inexpensive pH indicator strips similar to what we used in chemistry class.

We can test our saliva or urine with the same kit. Most of the time, our saliva test results will change with the time of day. Our morning urine may show acidity, but it depends on what, how, and when we eat and our hydration.

119   Ibid.

If we become dehydrated, just ate lunch, or maybe used an alcohol-based mouth rinse, it will affect our mouth's pH. Our mouth should test pH neutral. And when I test a patient with a pH strip, I do it to myself as a baseline. I know mine will test more pH neutral. This raises the credibility of the test and increases awareness of the potential problem. That's the psychology of using a test strip. If it's acidic, I know we have a problem.

Prebiotics and Probiotics

Prebiotics feed the good bacteria in your stomach. Probiotics try to improve the bacterial balance. I use a spore-based probiotic. There's also a way to take oral probiotics. Oral probiotics can also improve the bacteria, limit the overgrowth of the pathologic bacteria, and bring it back into balance. We always have good and bad bacteria in our bodies. We have the opportunity to keep it balanced.

When I examine a patient struggling with bleeding gums, I don't need much testing to determine my first response. I do my periodontal probing, and if I have bleeding, inflammation, and bone loss, I know there's active decay, active pathology, and periodontal disease. Then I have to educate the patient on that. We can't just attack it from the mouth; we have to attack it from the stomach and the gut.

Initially, I ask them to do a three-day diet journal, come in and discuss it. If I need to do something a little bit more with weight loss, I'll most likely send them to a naturopath, and we will work collaboratively. If they're having digestive problems, there's something out of balance. They might go to their physician for those stomach ailments and come out with a prescription for an antibiotic. But I only use antibiotics in dire situations because we know that taking antibiotics changes the bacteria. It's like a bomb, a bomb that's going to take out both the good and the harmful bacteria.

We do use antibiotics, reluctantly. With Lyme disease issues, or if we have a patient with a tooth abscess or some current infection, every time they take an antibiotic, it disrupts their gut microbiome negatively.

I suggest a probiotic during and immediately following antibiotic treatment to repopulate their stomach with some good stuff. After they stop antibiotics, they must take a good six to eight weeks of probiotics.

It's messy.

"And That's a Fine Kettle of Fish ..."

An old Scottish proverb goes, "That's a fine kettle of fish," made famous by the classic comedy team Laurel and Hardy in their films *Thicker Than Water* and *The Fixer-Uppers*. "Well, here's another nice kettle of fish you pickled me in!" A messy predicament.

This term comes from a Scottish custom of holding a waterside picnic, a "kettle of fish," where freshly caught live salmon are thrown into a kettle boiling over an open fire and then eaten out of hand.[120] Definitely a messy procedure. In its original form, the catchphrase was fittingly used as the last line of dialogue in the duo's last film in 1951, all classic and all well before my time.

In my closing thoughts in the following brief chapter, I tell a few fish stories that are not so messy. This may stimulate your *curiosity*, an attribute that brought us together in the first place.

---

120   Pascal Tréguer, "The Authentic Origin of 'a Pretty Kettle of Fish,'" https://wordhistories.net/ (Word Histories, June 2021), https://wordhistories.net/2016/07/06/kettle-of-fish/.

THE LIMITED WORLD OF DENTAL BENEFITS IN THE US

Think about your investment in oral health for a moment. Do you have mercury amalgam metals in your mouth? Do you have gold or other alloys in there interacting? Facing a wisdom tooth removal? Poor sleep? Poor diet? I hope not, but your dental insurance will likely not robustly cover these issues. But for many dental patients, if it exceeds the insurance maximum, they're done for the year. Many will even skip a cleaning if they have gone over their limit. That reduces their chances of maintaining optimal dental health and sustaining it.

WebMD observes that 77 percent of Americans have dental benefits, the National Association of Dental Plans says. Most people have private coverage, usually from an employer or group program. Large employers typically offer better dental benefits than small employers, and high-wage workers are more likely to receive them than low-wage workers. Medicare doesn't cover dental care, and most state Medicaid programs cover dental care only for children.

"To make the most of your benefits, you need to know these things."[121]

"When shopping for insurance, WebMD advises, you may see the term *dental benefits*, which is different from *insurance*."

"An *insurance plan* is meant to absorb risk—the risk that you'll need to have a tooth pulled, for instance, or to get a root canal—and covers costs accordingly. A *benefits plan* covers some things in total, but other things only partially, and others not at all. It's meant to be helpful, but it's not a catch-all," WebMD advises.

Folks should understand that dental insurance is not like medical insurance.

It's a valuable, helpful benefit. And it's also excellent for maintaining dental health, but it's not very practical for *restoring* somebody's dental health. Experts design dental insurance to keep you healthy, but when you start slipping, you may have some reimbursement. But if you let it

---

121 Kate Ashford, "Dental Insurance Plans: What's Covered, What's Not," webmd.com (WebMD, June 16, 2020), https://www.webmd.com/health-insurance/dental-insurance-overview#1.

slip too fast, too much, to get back to dental health, dental insurance can be very minimal. Folks need to understand that.

It's a shame that dental care is still an afterthought and must be mostly purchased separately from "health" insurance offerings.

If we all limit our dental care decisions to just what the benefits administrators allow, we're not getting the best dentistry has to offer. You may find that the benefits companies limit the optimal treatment for patients by delaying payments or denying predeterminations of services. *The tooth hasn't reached a threshold; the patient's not missing enough teeth to warrant a procedure.*

Such restrictions limit my philosophy of ideal dental health for everybody. In a perfect world, a medical insurance policy should fully cover the medical expenses of the mouth as well as every other part of the body. Because what happens in our mouth affects everything in the human body, taking good care of your teeth and gums avoids major health catastrophes down the road. Perhaps our insurance colleagues will one day discover that it's in their enlightened self-interest to cover the entire human body.

CHAPTER 11:

PARTING WORDS AND FISHING

The Power of a Receptive, Open Mind

Many men go fishing all of their lives without
knowing that it is not fish they are after.

—HENRY DAVID THOREAU

I want to leave you, dear reader, with some parting thoughts. By reading *Biologic Dentistry and a Better You* to this denouement, I suggest that you have an open mind, and open-mindedness is often missing in our culture. I applaud your curiosity.

Chasing our curiosity is what brought us together.

My willingness to question everything springs from being open to change and unusually curious about everything. In my final words to you, I wish to underscore just how wonderful that sense of curiosity and openness to new ideas has been in my journey.

I hope you understand that the landscape has changed in dentistry. Today there are dentists out there, probably in your community or nearby, that want to not only restore your teeth but help restore or improve your health. Dentistry is not a standalone anymore. Biologic dentistry recognizes the connections to organs of the human body. It's just separated medically and insurance-wise.

Embrace it fully with an open mind. Many folks think *all is okay* in their mouth, but in fact, likely not. This biologic approach to dentistry can improve their health. We're just not doing fillings, crowns, and cleanings. Things are progressing quickly.

I have always believed that healthcare providers must be passionate advocates for our patients. We have to stay relatively centered, but we need openness. Dental school rarely teaches this. We must learn it through trial and error; something must hit home deep.

I began my journey into biologic dentistry by applying my curiosity, experience, and instincts to my health struggles and those of my own family. That gave me the confidence to offer the same problem-solving approach to all my patients. I would never provide any holistic practice to my patients that I would not do myself.

When I worked full-time as an engineer early in my career, I would take the 6:20 a.m. train for an eighty-minute ride to work. At the end of those days, I would also attend night school, working on my master's in business. I kept up this pace for several years. *Ah, youth.*

And then, I left my job and went to dental school. My days were filled with education, always doing classwork, homework, or reading. Lifelong learning has just been the musical score of my life, my whole life, a soaring overture, by the way.

Chasing My Curiosity .

My life has been sweetened by my absolute love of my family and dentistry. Wherever curiosity leads, I find innovations worldwide with biologic dentistry and the oral-mouth systemic relationship. I try to do the best I can for the people who see me, and I have become someone people seek to solve problems, folks who have complicated issues. I don't run away from problems. I accept them. And I find that, almost weekly, my assistant can hear me muttering something like ... *Boy, this is not very easy to do. This isn't very easy, and I'm glad I can do it.* If my patient hears that mumbling self-talk, I usually cannot hide my smile because when they hear me say that, they know they're in the right spot.

I am not just glad to have the opportunity to solve difficult diagnostic dilemmas; I am thrilled. Once-new ideas have become commonplace today, and I reside on that leading edge with my biologic dentistry colleagues.

I have landed in my comfort zone. Not everybody does what I do or can do what I do. And that's not bragging; all clinicians who love their work feel that way. That confidence arises from experience. We need the challenges. We attract what we put out there. Patients come to me that need somebody close to them in their geographic orbit on whom they can count for help when the time comes. These patients, for the most part, are open-minded. They love biological techniques like drawing patients' blood before extractions and using PRF in place of synthetic materials for graphs to help the bone. They love the careful use of 3D x-ray CT scanning, the use of ozone, the elimination of mercury, and our minimalist philosophy. They cannot get enough of it. These folks do not want to put anything artificial in their bodies.

Sometimes, my rewards come walking in the door. I extracted two teeth from a patient recently, and she unexpectedly came back, asking me what more she could do. And I said, *What are you trying to accomplish? Why are you doing this? What are you trying to do?* She looked at me, smiled, and said, "Because I'm feeling so much better. I want to make sure I get it all." And that made me happy. That made me smile inside.

I am still intrigued by my observations. Always curious, I see things others may miss. For instance, I have provided dental care for patients with active breast cancer. And out of that curiosity, I will inquire, especially with a new patient, about any dental work. I will look at the x-rays and how much dental work they've had on that meridian side affected by the cancer. Then I'll investigate for any hidden source of infection that could be draining down through the lymphatic system with the possibility of affecting the breast cancer or possibly contributing to the cause or growth of that cancer.

We can test the teeth for vitality. We can investigate deep below the tooth to see if there are hidden infections, and if so, they could drain down the lymphatic system. We can use thermography technology to determine if that infection is spreading. This is an easy procedure to determine if oral infections are draining down your neck.

AT THIS POINT, I HOPE YOU ARE ASKING YOURSELF, "AM I GETTING THE BEST DENTISTRY I CAN GET?"

Thermography is an underutilized non-radiation imaging done with thermal cameras, another tool in my biologic dental toolbox.

At this point, I hope you are asking yourself, *Am I getting the best dentistry I can get?*

But there is a lack of universal access to clinical problem-solving in our medical culture. We all go to a superbly trained family doctor, who, faced with a long list of daily and urgent and complex patients, sends us to a specialist for GI problems, blood pressure issues, pain management, orthopedics, emotional issues, chronic disease management, allergies, and symptoms of unknown causes.

People come into our office regularly, frustrated that they're not getting the answers they need, a proper diagnosis. Folks sometimes feel they are hitting a dead end. Many are frustrated with the present system and access to solutions. Parents try to be informed advocates for their kids. What are they supposed to do? How are they supposed to be their advocate if they don't know where to turn? Armed with "Dr. Google," they do the best they can. You get a headache, *look it up*, and see brain tumor symptoms.

Our organs, our systems, are not independent of one another. Medicine today has become so complex that we must divide up specialization because of the breathtaking speed with which discoveries are made. We do not have the beloved country doctor coming to the house with the black bag. And those were the golden doctors, people with broad and diverse experience. They knew their patients well because they went to church with them, or their kids went to the same school. Folks had the same primary care doctor for years and years. Yes, if I had coronary disease, I would want a very skilled surgeon, of course. But a side effect of the rising demand on primary care providers is that their gatekeeper role has replaced a lot of good old-fashioned problem-solving.

Unfortunately, our present healthcare scheme in the USA operates in what many describe as an immoral status quo, with corporations profiting off of *financing* being a deciding factor for healthcare decisions. This has become increasingly hard to take from a dentist's point of view because we are now powerfully alert and observant of oral connections with the entire body. Our services have not yet made the radar screen of big business health insurance providers.

Biologic dentistry can often provide many answers because we study the mouth for connections and clues. Periodontal disease can be a significant factor in systemic inflammation. We notice sleep patterns, speech patterns, breathing, bruxing, and toxic metal issues. We use advanced imaging and holistic surgical techniques. We might even glance at the voltage in your body or use laser technology or ozone to make you better. People who experience this advanced care don't want to go back, and they have become, well, more open-minded. Your oral care, more than just the ongoing health of your teeth, represents your entire health picture. As a scientist and a dentist, I see advancements such as these constantly emerging. And if we do not stay abreast of this stuff, then we're not doing our job. If, for instance, we paid no attention to the brilliant research of Dr. Maiken Nedergaard, we would not place so much emphasis on the power of sleep and the importance of detoxing the brain.

Conformity

Usually, open-minded folks resist conformity. I have no problem with some of my colleagues saying, *He is a little bit out there*. Not at all. I like that. I am not a conformist for the most part. I drive between the lines, questioning everything, but I safely veer outside those lines from time to time. This has been important to me as our clinical world has actually gotten narrower and veering outside those lines provides better care.

To those who brush all this aside and become critical, okay. That's your right. But if you consider just relaxing a little bit and trying to be open-minded a bit more, there's a whole world of innovative care awaiting you.

I pay attention to those whose ideas are on the edges and lead from out front. I don't go looking for serious dental problems, they find me, and I don't do dentistry that people don't need because I don't need that headache.

Can-You-Believe-It's-Real Moments

A good friend of mine noted that he fully understands *why* I love to go fishing. He reminded me of the essence of fishing—to seek and find the fish and then solve the problem of how to catch them and have an open mind about it all.

It's my hobby and my break from the office. Immersing myself fully in the fantastic nature of the planet re-energizes me continually. I had never really thought about why I liked to fish. I just always have thoroughly enjoyed this avocation. And if I must admit, I am pretty good at it. There's a sudden and miraculous grace to the moment of a big strike, and in fact, to every moment getting to that encounter.

No wonder you like fishing, my friend said. *That's who you are: stubbornly curious, intensely observative, and motivated by problem-solving.*

He's right. It's the can-you-believe-it's-real moments of tossing a line into the water surrounded by the most beautiful mountains on earth. We listen to the environment's clues, noting weather, the water temperature, the speed of the water, tributary inlets, the time of day, the eddies and turbulence, the shadows, the vegetation, observing their subtler "bow wakes" or their graceful acrobatic jumps for bugs, the depth at which you get unexpected strikes on your lure or fly.

My dad taught me to fish. Many years later, I brought him to the Orvis School to learn fly fishing, and then we fished for striped bass off Cape Cod, and soon after, we went to the streams out west. A powerful father-son experience to go out with him today; it's now my turn to teach him. I have many beautiful memories, but probably the best fishing trip ever was when we floated the Yellowstone River about twenty years ago.

My father and I fished the Madison River, which runs 140 miles through stunning scenery; we fished twelve miles of the Gallatin River, which runs through Wyoming and Montana. We fished a few smaller rivers in the park, culminating with that highlight reel float trip down Yellowstone. The Yellowstone River stretches 678 miles, the longest free-flowing river in the continental US.

Fly fishing the Yellowstone in the summer is best about an hour before sunset. The river explodes with surfacing trout, many leaving the water completely. On this day, the sky was metallic blue, hinting at a deep orange/puce sunset show, framing this gorgeous cold mountain river on a hot summer day. The current was moving us fast. Fly fishing from a drift boat, we caught rainbow, brown, and cutthroat trout left and right.

We had never caught so many fish per mile. (Advanced anglers measure rivers in *fish per mile* of river.) That was an epic trip for me because it was early in my father's boat fly fishing career. He was transitioning from "walking and wading" to learning to fly fish from a drift boat. Decades ago, he taught me how to fish, and now, I was teaching him how to fly fish while floating down the river, one of those moments you know you will never forget. And he had a smile on his face as big as a Cheshire cat, as you can imagine, thinking that he was catching the greatest number of fish in his life. He was.

We later had another kind of *A River Runs Through It* moment out in Colorado near Breckenridge, where I caught a twenty-four-inch rainbow trout. I vividly remember the altitude catching up to both of us. And I worked for about thirty minutes to get her to the shore to release her. And that was like, my golly, that thing was a monster. She was jumping, twisting, and somehow, I managed to hold onto her and barely keep her in the net. That was my biggest trout. Releasing that giant was a great moment. We catch and holistically release every fish.

I share this story because there are many correlations between the art of fishing and the art of being a biologic dentist, the way you practice it, the deliberateness, the heightened senses, and the passion for it. There are a lot of parallels there.

You have to understand the stream and the flow rate holistically. It's not going down the river and putting a worm on a bobber. There's a lot to it. There's the entomology of it, trying to match the hatch and understanding the techniques. It's quite technical, with a great deal of reliance on observation, just like biologic dentistry.

We asked the other anglers on the river: *Having any luck?* (Well, where I fish, luck has little to do with it.) *What's working for ya?*

I get the same deep, inner personal satisfaction solving the problem of catching a clever, elusive rainbow trout as I do when we solve a patient's difficult diagnostic dilemma with biologic and holistic methods, using the same powers of observation and problem-solving mentality.

I don't keep trophies of my successful fishing adventures. Most of my dance partners are probably out there still swimming today.

I tune into a deeper spiritual channel out there. I can recalibrate in the wilderness.

The fishing avocation to which I now admit full addiction is made even better by the "catch and release" philosophy, using barbless hooks and holistically returning the fish to the water in the midst of this hallucinatory beauty to be caught again and perhaps spread the news far and wide throughout the water, that these hooks "ain't so bad."

And then there is always an obligatory sharing of what we learned this day with other anglers on the river, hoping they can match our luck, and then later, anyone else who will not cringe when I begin to tell a fish story.

Rob Herzog, DDS

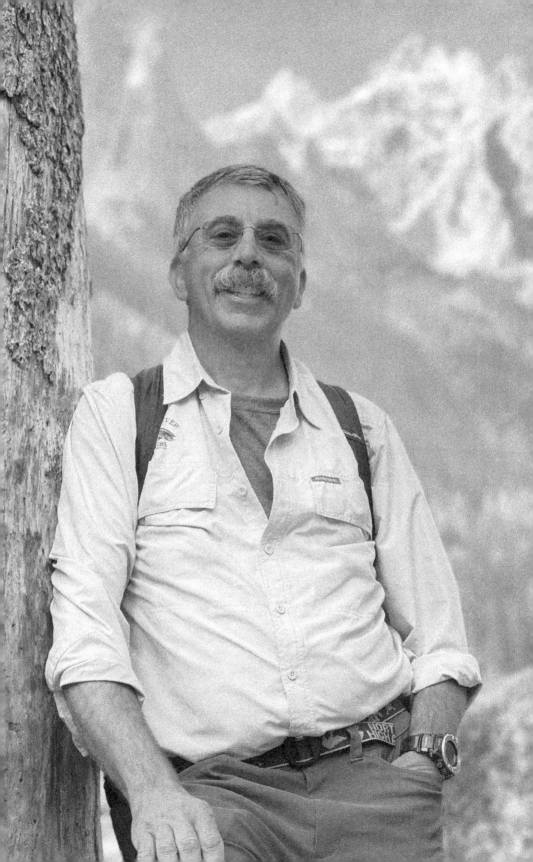

DR. ROBERT HERZOG, DDS, FAGD

Certified naturopathic and biological dentist, NMD, IBDM.

A certified SMART dentist.

Fellow of the Academy of General Dentistry (FAGD).

Accredited Member of the International Association of Oral Medicine and Toxicology.

University of Buffalo School of Dental Medicine.

Board certified in integrative biologic dental medicine by the American Board of Integrative Medicine and Dentistry.

Certified by the American Naturopathic Medical Association as a naturopathic physician/dentist.

Certified in ozone therapy from the American College of Integrative Medicine and Dentistry.

Master of science in management technology at Polytechnic University.

Bachelor of electrical engineering at SUNY Maritime College.

Dental residency at the Albany Veterans Hospital.

Member of the American Dental Association, the State Dental Society of New York.

Dawson Academy scholar.

Member of the International Academy of Mini Dental Implants.

Military Experience: US Naval Reserve, Strategic Sealift Officer, licensed merchant mariner.

Dr. Herzog enjoys all aspects of general dentistry, particularly prosthetic dentistry (implants, crowns, bridges, and dentures) and oral surgery. He finds cosmetic and aesthetic dentistry especially rewarding as it often changes the quality of life for his patients. He places zirconia, titanium implants, and mini implants to improve the comfort of partials or dentures. Dr. Herzog also recommends the safe removal of mercury amalgam fillings according to the International Academy of Oral Medicine and Toxicology (IAOMT) protocol.

Dr. Herzog has been recognized as Citizen of the Year and honored by News Channel 13, St. Peter's Health Care Services, and the *Times Union* as a Jefferson Award recipient for service to his community.

He was honored multiple times as America's Best Dentists, America's Top Dentists, New York's Top Dentists, and one of Albany's Top Dentists as selected by his dental peers and published in the *Capital Region Living* magazine.

His other passions include spending time with his family and most outdoor activities such as fishing, canoeing, hiking, snowshoeing, and national parks. He serves as a New York State Licensed Outdoor Guide. Dr. Herzog has been a leader in the Boy Scouts of America for thirty years, one of thirteen Eagle Scouts in his family dating from the 1960s to the present. Through the decades of being a scout leader, he and his wife Susan have helped young people achieve their potential of becoming Eagle Scouts, including his three boys, Luke, Brian, and Eric.